INTERMITTENT FASTING 101

For Beginners. Burn Fat Quickly With The 101 Methods, Eat The Foods You Love In a Healthy Way. Includes 5/2 Method To Maximize Weight Loss.

Table of Contents

INTRODUCTION 8

CHAPTER ONE: INTERMITTENT FASTING 10

    WHAT IS INTERMITTENT FASTING?   10

    WHO SHOULD OR SHOULD NOT TRY INTERMITTENT FASTING? 11

    POSSIBLE HEALTH BENEFITS OF INTERMITTENT FASTING 15

CHAPTER TWO: TIPS FOR MOTIVATION AND SUCCESS 22

    12 FASTING TIPS THAT WILL HELP YOU REALLY LOSE WEIGHT 22

    HOW TO BEGIN INTERMITTENT FASTING IN 5 NON-INTIMIDATING STEPS 28

CHAPTER THREE: EXERCISING AND EATING RIGHT FOR A HEALTHY LIFESTYLE 37

    REASONS TO EXERCISE AND EAT RIGHT APART FROM WEIGHT LOSS 44

    THE BEST REASONS TO BREAK A SWEAT 45

    THE BEST REASONS TO START HEALTHY EATING 54

CHAPTER FOUR: TYPES OF INTERMITTENT FASTING 62

    5:2 INTERMITTENT FASTING AKA. THE FAST DIET 62

    INTERMITTENT FASTING 16/8   63

    THE 24-HOUR FAST (24 HOURS FAST ONCE A WEEK) 66

20/4 INTERMITTENT FASTING A.K.A. WARRIOR DIET 67

THE 36/12 HOURS FAST (ALTERNATE DAY FAST) 69

23/1 INTERMITTENT FASTING AKA ONE MEAL A DAY 71

CIRCADIAN RHYTHM FASTING 71

PROLONGED A.K.A EXTENDED FASTING 72

CHAPTER FIVE: INTERMITTENT FASTING FOR WEIGHT LOSS....73

HOW DOES INTERMITTENT FASTING AFFECT YOUR HORMONES? 73

INTERMITTENT FASTING HELPS YOU LOSE WEIGHT AND REDUCE CALORIES 74

HOW EXACTLY DOES INTERMITTENT FASTING WORK FOR WEIGHT LOSS? 75

REASONS YOU ARE NOT LOSING WEIGHT WHILE DOING INTERMITTENT FASTING 77

HOW TO SUCCEED WITH INTERMITTENT FASTING PROTOCOL 83

CHAPTER SIX: THE 5:2 METHOD STEP BY STEP............ 88

WHAT IS THE 5:2 FAST DIET? 88

CAN THE 5:2 FAST DIET HELP YOU LOSE WEIGHT? 88

IS THE 5:2 FAST DIET GOOD FOR YOUR HEALTH? 89

IS THE 5:2 DIET SUSTAINABLE FOR LONG-TERM WEIGHT LOSS? 90

WHAT YOU CAN AND CANNOT EAT ON THE 5:2 FAST DIET 91

WHEN YOU SHOULD OR SHOULD NOT FAST ON THE 5:2 DIET   96

WHO MUST NOT TRY THE 5:2 DIET?   97

EXERCISE ON THE 5:2 FAST DIET   98

OTHER HEALTH BENEFITS OF THE 5:2 DIET   102

CHAPTER SEVEN: 5:2 FASTING DAY RECIPES 106

PARMESAN EGG TOAST WITH TOMATOES   106

GREEK BREAKFAST WRAPS   107

CURRIED CHICKEN BREAST WRAPS   108

PROTEIN POWER SWEET POTATOES   109

BAKED SALMON FILLETS WITH TOMATO AND MUSHROOMS   110

AVOCADO AND FENNEL SALAD WITH BALSAMIC VINAIGRETTE   111

HEARTY SHRIMP AND KALE SOUP   112

PENNE PASTA WITH VEGETABLES   114

PORK LOIN CHOPS WITH MANGO SALSA   115

SPINACH AND SWISS CHEESE OMELETTE   116

LEMON-SESAME CHICKEN AND ASPARAGUS   118

GRILLED CHICKEN SALAD WITH POPPY SEED SAUCE   119

TOASTED PEPPER JACK SANDWICHES   120

BROILED HALIBUT WITH GARLIC SPINACH   121

QUICK MISO SOUP WITH SHRIMP AND BOK CHOY   122

QUINOA WITH SWEET POTATOES AND CURRIED BLACK BEANS   123

CHAPTER EIGHT: HEALTHY RECIPES FOR NON-FASTING DAYS **126**

   BREAKFAST   126

      SALMON AND TOMATO EGG SANDWICHES   126

      NUTTY PEACH PARFAITS   127

      COCOA-BANANA BREAKFAST SMOOTHIE   128

      SCRAMBLED EGG SOFT TACOS 129

      CRANBERRY-WALNUT WHOLE WHEAT PANCAKES   130

      HERB AND SWISS FRITTATA   131

      SCRAMBLED EGGS WITH MUSHROOMS AND ONIONS   132

      VANILLA-ALMOND PROTEIN SHAKE   133

      GRILLED FRUIT SALAD 134

      EASY GRANOLA BARS   135

      HEARTY HOT CEREAL WITH BERRIES   136

      PECAN-BANANA POPS 137

   LUNCH   139

      TUNA AND BEAN SALAD POCKETS   139

      SHRIMP AND CRANBERRY SALAD   140

      CHICKEN BREAST WITH ROASTED SUMMER VEGGIES   141

      SEAFOOD-STUFFED AVOCADOES   142

      EASY CHICKEN PASTA SOUP   144

      CHOPPED BLT SALAD   145

      TOASTED HAM, SWISS, AND ARUGULA SANDWICHES   146

      POWER-PACKED GREEN SMOOTHIE   147

QUICK AND LIGHT WHITE BEAN CHILI   148

EGGPLANT, HUMMUS, AND GOAT CHEESE SANDWICHES   149

VEGETABLE MARKET SCRAMBLE   150

DINNER   151

TANGY ORANGE CHICKEN BREAST   151

GRILLED SHRIMP AND BLACK BEAN SALAD 153

MUSTARD-MAPLE-GLAZED SALMON   154

TUSCAN-STYLE BAKED SEA BASS   155

PORTOBELLO CHEESEBURGERS   156

FLANK STEAK SPINACH SALAD   158

CHICKEN PICADILLO   159

CHICKEN FLORENTINE-STYLE 160

EASY BLACK BEAN SOUP   162

HEARTY VEGETABLE SOUP   163

MUSHROOM-STUFFED ZUCCHINI   164

ZESTY BEEF KABOBS   165

CONCLUSION.. **168**

INTRODUCTION

One of the most commonly-known health trends is intermittent fasting (IF), which involves alternating cycles of eating and fasting (starvation).

Many individuals practice fasting as part of their religion or in preparation for some kind of spiritual experience. Others use fasting to periodically cleanse their bodies of accumulated waste and toxins. Some people claim that periodic short fasts increase concentration and clear their minds.

Fasting has also been used by many individuals as a way to lose body fat and weight. This reason we fast has become extremely popular in recent years. This is in part because of many books and websites that promote fasting as a weight-loss strategy.

There are as several types of fasting diets as there are many reasons for fasting. Some are long term weight management plans and some are short term solutions. Although, there are healthier versions of intermittent fasting plans, many are far from being healthy in terms of nutrition. These diets typically recommend long-term fasting, encourage dieters to eat whatever they want on non-fast days, or lack guidelines that will assist the follower make good nutritional decisions in the future.

The 5: 2 method for maximizing weight loss is an intermittent fasting plan that encourages followers to eat plenty of wholes, nutritious foods on both fast and non-fasting days. Along with being a healthier alternative to some popular fasting diets, it's also much easier (and more enjoyable) to follow than some of the more extreme intermittent fasting diets.

Losing weight and body fat isn't all about looking good temporarily; it is about feeling good, learning to eat healthily and in a sustainable way and improving one's health and quality of life in general. This is the mission of **Intermittent Fasting 101.**

The purpose of this beginner's guide is to provide everything you need to know about intermittent fasting to get started.

CHAPTER ONE: INTERMITTENT FASTING

Intermittent fasting is all about alternating between periods of fasting and eating, and has recently become very popular. Not only was it the "most modern" weight loss search term in 2020, it was also introduced in the New England Journal of Medicine review article.

Intermittent fasting can offer significant health benefits when done correctly, including weight loss, reversing type 2 diabetes, and many other things. Additionally, it can save you time and money.

WHAT IS INTERMITTENT FASTING?

Intermittent fasting – is that any different from starving oneself?

Yes. Fasting is different from starvation in one vital way: control. Starvation is the involuntary unavailability of food for a long time. It can lead to great suffering or even death. It is neither controlled nor deliberate.

In another way, fasting is the voluntary abstention from food for spiritual, health or other reasons. It is performed by a person who is not underweight and has enough stored body fat to live. If done correctly, fasting should not cause suffering and certainly never death.

Food is readily accessible, but we decide not to eat it. We may decide to do this for any period of time, from a few hours to a few days or – though with medical supervision - up to a week or more. You can start a fast at any time you want and you can also end a fast whenever you want.

Whenever you don't eat, you are fasting intermittently. For example, you can fast between dinner and breakfast the next day, for a period of about 12 to 2 hours. In this sense, intermittent fasting should be seen as part of everyday life.

Consider the term "breakfast." It refers to the meal that interrupts the fast, which is done daily.

Instead of being some sort of unusual and cruel punishment, the English language implicitly recognizes that fasting must be done daily, even if only for a short time.

Intermittent fasting is not uncommon, but it is a part of everyday and normal life. It is perhaps the most powerful and oldest dietary intervention imaginable. However, one way or another, we lose its power and neglect its therapeutic potential. Learning to fast properly gives us the option to use it or not.

WHO SHOULD OR SHOULD NOT TRY INTERMITTENT FASTING?

While intermittent fasting has worked for me, it isn't for everyone. First, intermittent fasting isn't just another way of saying "free ride." Randomly skipping meals while you continue to follow a diet rich in processed foods won't help you lose fat and improve your health.

So, while there is no "appropriate" way to practice fasting, any decent protocol will require some attention to nutritional specifications. You must be prepared to do this work.

Some people will find intermittent fasting very uncomfortable or irritating to practice. And for others, their risks far outweigh the potential benefits. In fact, for some individuals, intermittent fasting can be quite dangerous.

Before you skip your next meal, you'll probably want to know if you fall into this category.

Here are the details, based on several case studies and a small amount of published research.

Intermittent Fasting: Green Light

In my experience, it's very likely that you will be successful with intermittent fasting if:

- You are already an experienced athlete
- You have a history of monitoring calories and food intake (for example, you have "dieted" before)
- You have no children or you are single
- Your job allows you to experience periods of underperformance as you adjust to a new plan
- Your partner (if you have one) is very supportive
- You are a man

The first five factors will make it easier for you to incorporate protocols into your lifestyle, while the final condition (being a man) seems to affect the results.

Intermittent fasting: Yellow Light

In the meantime, if you meet the following criteria, proceed with caution:

- You have performance-oriented or customer-oriented jobs
- You have children or you are married
- You compete in athletics/sport
- You are a woman

Again, the first three conditions make tracking intermittent fasting protocols much more difficult and may make it impossible for you. Additionally, trying to fast can conflict with your sport's performance goals.

Regarding the latter condition, some researchers suggest that fasting causes insomnia, anxiety, irregular periods, and other indications of hormonal deregulation in women.

In particular, women seem to get worse with more severe forms of intermittent fasting than men. Therefore, if you are female and want to give fasting a try, I recommend that you start with a very relaxed approach.

Intermittent Fasting: Red Light

Finally, there are some people who absolutely shouldn't be concerned with intermittent fasting. Do not try intermittent fasting if:

- You have a history of eating disorders
- You are pregnant
- You are chronically stressed
- You are new to diet and exercise

- You sleep badly

If you're new to exercise and diet, intermittent fasting may seem like a magic bullet for weight loss. But you would be much smarter to deal with any nutritional deficiencies before you start experimenting with fasting. Make sure you start with a solid nutritional platform.

Pregnant women need extra energy, so if you are starting a family, now is not the time you should fast.

Ditto if you don't sleep and/or you are under chronic stress. Your body needs nutrition, not extra stress. And if you've had eating disorder issues in the past, you probably recognize that a fasting protocol can take you down a path that can create more problems for you. Why toil with your health? You can get similar benefits in other ways.

So intermittent fasting does not suit you? How do you get in shape without trying intermittent fasting?

How can you lose weight and get in shape if intermittent fasting isn't a good option for you?

Learn the basics of good nutrition. It is by far the best thing you can do for your health and fitness.

Cook and eat whole foods. Regularly exercise. Be consistent. And if you want help with all of that, find a mentor or coach. The last part is relevant, even if you decide to try intermittent fasting.

While self-experimentation is good, guided experimentation is even better. Especially when it is supervised by an experienced technician.

POSSIBLE HEALTH BENEFITS OF INTERMITTENT FASTING

Intermittent fasting has received a lot of praise for its potential effect on our body weight and some other health parameters, but should you believe it?

Intermittent fasting (IF), one of the most talked about diets today, is a form of eating that denotes periods of time for food and fasting. And there is no sign that interest is decreasing.

There are a few several approaches, but the two most common are 16: 8, which requires you to squeeze all meals of the day into an eight-hour window and fast for the rest of the 16 hours, and 5:2, where we spent five days of the week eating normally and two for fasting (generally defined as eating only 500-600 calories per day).

Why would someone choose this way of eating instead of a standard diet like low carb or fat? Some say that fasting has many health benefits. So far, research has shown the benefits of intermittent fasting to the point that it is worth it as a method of weight loss, blood sugar control, and slowing the aging process.

So, instead of looking at the affirmations at face value, we decided to dive into them and explore if the science doesn't yet stack up or if the ten benefits proclaimed by intermittent fasting are legitimate.

1. Weight loss

Most individuals start intermittent fasting to lose weight. And that statement seems to hold up, at least in the short term. It is possible that any version of intermittent fasting can contribute to the loss of weight. The researchers analyzed data from 13 studies and found that the average weight loss ranged from 1.3% for a two-week trial to 8% for an eight-week trial.

This is probably good news if you're hoping to lose weight through fasting, but the fact that these studies were short term means it's hard to know if intermittent fasting is sustainable and can help you shed those pounds off for a long term.

Another catch: The amount of weight lost doesn't seem to be more than you'd expect from any other low-calorie diet, and depending on how many calories you eat each day, you may even gain weight. After all, the diet does not limit high calorie foods.

When the diet is done correctly, intermittent fasting can be as effective as regular calorie restriction. Some individuals, especially busy people who don't have time to plan their meals, may even find a time-limited diet easier to follow than something like the keto diet or the paleo diet.

2. Lowering blood pressure

Intermittent fasting can help reduce high blood pressure within the short term. A study issued in June 2018 in Nutrition and Healthy Aging found that 16:8 significantly reduced systolic blood pressure in 23 study participants. The link has been shown in animal and human studies. Additionally, an October 2019 study published in the European Journal of Nutrition found that intermittent fasting resulted in even greater drops in systolic blood pressure than another diet that did not have set meal times.

Having healthy blood pressure is important: harmful levels can increase your risk for heart disease, stroke, and kidney disease.

But studies so far show that these blood pressure benefits only last while you practice intermittent fasting. After the diet was over and people resumed eating normally, the researchers found that the blood pressure readings returned to baseline levels.

3. Reduction of inflammation

Animal studies have shown that intermittent fasting and general calorie restriction can reduce levels of inflammation, although clinical trials are scarce. The authors of a study issued in Nutrition Research wanted to know if this link also exists in humans. The study involved 50 participants who fasted on Ramadan, the Muslim holiday, which involves fasting from sunrise to sunset and eating at night. The study presented that during the period of fasting, pro-inflammatory markers were lower than normal, as were blood pressure, body fat, and body weight.

4. Lower cholesterol

A two-day fast can help lower total cholesterol and LDL cholesterol when done in conjunction with resistance exercise. LDL cholesterol is the "evil" cholesterol that can increase the risk of stroke or heart disease, according to the CDCP. Obesity researchers also noted that intermittent fasting reduces the presence of triglycerides, which are fats in the blood that can cause stroke, heart attack, or heart disease. A caveat here: The study was short, so more research is needed to understand whether the effects of intermittent fasting on cholesterol are lasting.

5. Better outcomes for stroke survivors

More healthy levels of cholesterol and the reduction of blood pressure (two benefits mentioned above) play a significant role in minimizing your risk of stroke. However, that is not the only stroke-related benefits of intermittent fasting. It has been found that intermittent fasting and reducing calories in general can provide a protective mechanism for the brain. In cases where a stroke does occur, it seems that eating this way pre-stroke can prevent brain damage. The researchers say that studies are needed in the future to determine if following intermittent fasting post-stroke can help recovery.

6. Improved brain function

Intermittent fasting can improve mental acuity and focus. And there is initial research to support this idea: A study on mice published in February 2018 found that it may help protect against age-related memory decline. Intermittent fasting can improve connections in the cerebral hippocampus and also protect against amyloid plaques, which are found in patients with Alzheimer's disease. This study was only conducted on animals, so it is not yet clear whether the benefit is true for humans.

7. Protection against cancer

Some studies have shown that fasting every other day can reduce the risk of cancer, reduce the development of lymphoma, limiting the survival of cancer and slow the spread of cancer cells. The studies that showed the benefit of cancer were all animal studies, however, and more studies are needed to understand the mechanism behind these effects and confirm a benefit for humans.

8. Increase in cell turnover

The period for resting involved in intermittent fasting maximizes autophagy, which is "an important bodily detoxification function for cleaning out damaged cells." In other words, a break in food and digestion gives the body a chance to heal itself and get rid of wastes inside cells that can speed up aging.

9. Reduced insulin resistance

It is suggested that intermittent fasting may help stabilize blood sugar levels in people with diabetes because it restores insulin, although more research is needed. The idea is that limiting calories may improve insulin resistance, which is a marker for type 2 diabetes. Fasting, like the type of fasting associated with intermittent fasting, encourages the reduction in insulin levels, which may play a role in reducing type 2 risk.

10. Reduced risk of cardiovascular problems

According to the nutrient study above, when insulin levels drop, the risk of dangerous cardiovascular events, such as congestive heart failure, decreases, which is vital for patients with type 2 diabetes as they are three to five times more susceptible to die from heart disease than grownups without diabetes.

While there are no studies in humans to confirm the benefit; Observational studies have shown that intermittent fasting can provide cardiovascular and metabolic benefits. It is suspected that changes in metabolic parameters, such as lowering triglyceride levels and lowering blood sugar, are the result of weight loss and would be achieved regardless of how the weight was lost, whether by intermittent fasting or a low-card diet, for example.

11. Greater longevity

Some animal and rodent studies have shown that intermittent fasting can prolong life, perhaps because fasting appears to increase resistance to age-related diseases. While these are promising results, it has been difficult to replicate them in human studies. Until that happens, you better be skeptical of this potential benefit.

12. A better night's sleep

If you've ever felt like you're in a coma after a big meal, you know that eating can affect wakefulness and drowsiness. Some followers of intermittent fasting report that they can sleep better by following this form of eating. "Intermittent fasting and mealtime can affect sleep. Why?

One theory is that intermittent fasting regulates the circadian rhythm, which controls sleep patterns. A regulated circadian rhythm implies you'll fall asleep and wake up easily, although research supporting this theory is limited.

The other theory focuses on the fact that having your last meal earlier in the evening means that you will have digested the food before you sleep. The digestion is better when upright and falling asleep with a full stomach can cause bedtime acid reflux or heartburn, which can interfere with sleep.

CHAPTER TWO: TIPS FOR MOTIVATION AND SUCCESS

Let's face it: dieting can be difficult. Following the one that involves fasting (yes, a situation where you won't eat)? Well it can be even more difficult. And for some, the thought of skipping a meal on purpose is enough to make them hungry, if not worse.

Even so, there are many people who are up to the challenge, not to mention people who has even seen serious results of a diet food structured and planned. So what's the secret to their success? Following at least one, if not all of these 12 tips for acing a fasting diet, directly from the nutritionist.

12 FASTING TIPS THAT WILL HELP YOU REALLY LOSE WEIGHT

1. Make your new meal plan easier.

While it can be alluring to jump right into your new eating routine (the initial excitement is real), it can be difficult and make you more hungry and uncomfortable. Instead, we recommend starting slowly, say, doing two or three days of intermittent fasting for the first week, and then "gradually increasing week by week." Taking it slowly, this is not only good advice for fasting, but good for life (just saying).

2. Know the difference between wanting to eat and needing to eat.

Once you hear your stomach snoring, you may feel like there is no way that you are going to go through X more amount of hours without food. Tune in that hunger signal. Ask yourself if hunger is boredom or real hunger. If you are bored, let yourself be distracted by another task.

If you are very hungry but don't feel faint or dizzy, drink hot mint tea, as mint is known to reduce appetite, or drink water to fill your stomach until the next meal.

Now, if you've been trying intermittent fasting for a while and still experience extreme hunger between periods, you need to think twice. You need to add more nutrient-dense or calorie-dense foods over the eight hour period or consider that this may not be the greatest plan for you. Add healthy fats such as peanut butter, avocado, nuts coconut and olive oil, as well as proteins during eating time can help you stay satisfied and satiated longer.

3. Eat as needed.

Technically, intense hunger and fatigue shouldn't occur when you follow the 16: 8 fasting method (perhaps the most common). But if you are feeling extremely dizzy, listen, because your body is likely to be trying to tell you something. You perhaps have low blood sugar and need something to eat, and repeat with me, okay.

By definition, fasting is about removing some, if not all, of food, so don't blame yourself for breaking the fast with small and smart bites. Your best bet? Choose a high-protein snack like a few slices of turkey breast, or a hard-boiled egg or two (to help you stay in a ketogenic (fat-burning) state). You can then revert to the fast, of course, if you wish.

4. Hydrate, hydrate, hydrate.

Even on an empty stomach, drinking water and beverages such as coffee and tea (without milk) are not only permitted, but, especially in the case of H2O, encouraged.

We recommend setting reminders throughout the day and especially during times of fasting to get plenty of fluids. Try to fill at least 2, if not 3 liters per day.

5. Break your fast slowly and steadily.

After several hours without eating, you can feel like a human vacuum cleaner ready to suck whatever is on your plate. But cooking in minutes isn't much of a problem for your body or waistline, research shows. Instead, you want to eat slowly and chew well to allow your digestive system to completely process the food. Also, it will help you in getting a better idea of your fullness, to avoid overeating

6. Avoid overeating.

By the way, just because you've stopped fasting doesn't mean you should be enjoying yourself. Overeating can not only make you feel bloated and uncomfortable, but it can also sabotage the weight loss goals that likely led you to intermittent fasting in the first place. In short: it is not necessarily the quantity of what is on your plate that can help you be satisfied longer, but what is on your plate. Which brings us to the next fasting tip ...

7. Keep your meals balanced.

Having a rich mix of protein, fiber, healthy fats and carbohydrates can help you is to lose weight and avoid hunger during fasting. A good example is a roasted chicken (you want about 4 to 6 oz of protein) with half a small sweet potato and spinach stew with garlic and olive oil.

As for fruits, it is advisable to choose those low index glycemic, which are digested, absorbed and metabolized, which result in a lower rise in blood sugar. A stable blood sugar level helps prevent food cravings and is therefore the key to successful weight loss.

8. Try out different schedules.

Although for the most part, I recommend 16: 8, But it is better to look at your overall lifestyle to see which fasting method is right for you.

For example, if you wake up early, we suggest you eat for the first few hours, say 10am. to 6pm., then quickly until the next morning at 10 a.m. The loveliness of intermittent fasting is that it can be easily changed and flexible according to you and your schedule.

Another option is to stop early and have breakfast later each day to gradually increase the strength of the fast. "We all naturally fast once a day while we sleep, so maybe you practice 'shutting down the kitchen' first." For instance, "close" the kitchen at 9 p.m. and stop eating until 8 a.m. for breakfast. It's a natural 11 hour fast! If desired, change these times slowly (for example, kitchen closes at 8 p.m., breakfast at 9 a.m.).

9. Avoid fasting for 24 hours.

We advise against fasting for a whole day, as it can "lead to increased weakness, hunger and food consumption and therefore weight gain."

If your goal is to lose weight, considering your overall calorie intake and working on the scale may be more beneficial than resisting fasting for a long time (especially if you are the type who drinks too much).

10. Adapt your exercise routine.

First thing's first: you can certainly exercise if you are on a fasting diet. But (!!) you want to know what types of movements you are doing and when. If you choose to exercise on an empty stomach, I recommend that you exercise early in the morning when you can have more energy.

That said, it is important to remember that if you are not adequately fueling your muscles, then you run a greater risk of injury. Therefore, you can consider low impact exercises like yoga or cardio at steady state in mornings on an empty stomach and book that hardcore class for after eating.

11. Track your journey.

Believe it or not, keeping a food journal can help you with your fasting regimen. A food journal for fasting?! Yes, you read that right. While you don't report as many meals, actively noting details like emotions and symptoms (level of hunger, weakness, etc.) that occur during intermittent fasting can help you gauge your progress. It can also help you notice trigger points that make it harder to fast, like drinking the night before.

12. Listen to your body.

That one is important. Always keep your eyes open for symptoms such as dizziness, fatigue, irritability (uncommon), headache, anxiety, and difficulty concentrating. If you have any of these challenges, consider breaking the fast. All of these are signs that the body is hungry and may need nutrition. And if you begin to feel colder than usual, that's even more of a sign to stop fasting.

Having said that, be patient. Your body might take few days to get used to fasting, and you might feel hungrier and weaker than normal. So don't lose your mind if you experience these (less severe) sensations for a week or more. If these challenges last longer, however, and symptoms like those with more than dizziness occur, we recommend that you drop the diet and find something else to help you reach your goals. There is no point in getting sick for any amount of pounds.

HOW TO BEGIN INTERMITTENT FASTING IN 5 NON-INTIMIDATING STEPS

It's scary, isn't it? What if there was a calm and safe way to start? What if your current abilities are sufficient?

It's like this:

Instead of seeing it as another difficult task that you owe to your health, have it as a personal experience.

- Break it down into small, step-by-step, but easily achievable actions that ensure completion.
- Or watch and analyze what you learn
- Draw your assumption: is fasting right for you?

So you are not committing to it, you are here to learn. Because, like most individuals, you learn by doing. Doesn't that already seem easier? But...

Before starting

Talk to your doctor before you start. Especially if you are on drugs or have a health problem. Stop if you feel bad.

Keep it simple. Fasting (in this experiment) is known as consuming only pure water (flat or carbonated), black coffee, or tea without sugar.

Keep it calm. Eat your usual meals during the meal window. In my personal experience, intermittent fasting is most effective when combined with a low-carb, high-fat diet with real whole foods. But throwing the perfect combination for the best results isn't your goal now ... it's to finish a fast.

The schedule (i.e. 7 p.m.) is mentioned for the sake of simplicity. You don't have to follow them. You may adjust the hours according to your schedule.

What days of the week? In my experience, weekday fasting is more convenient because it is more structured and has fewer variables. But that may not be applicable to you. What you are looking for are those days you are more likely to say, "Where's the time gone? I forgot to eat!"

Slip ups are okay. First of all, forgive yourself. You can start from day one or resume from where you stopped. Do whatever is easiest to get back on track. Then...

Focus on your goal

Why do you want to experience intermittent fasting? What's in intermittent fasting for you?

Weight loss, weight maintenance. Fasting decreases hormones such as insulin and increases HGH and norefinefrina, that make stored body fat more accessible to burn to produce the energy and lose fat.

Avoid drugs, relieve symptoms. Fasting helps prevent diabetes, heart disease, reduce inflammation.

Prevent serious illnesses, longevity. Studies show that fasting can provide protection against Alzheimer's cancer and can help you live longer.

Think about why you made this choice when you feel "deprived."

Solve your concerns

What makes you nervous about intermittent fasting that makes you quit?

It's okay to ditch breakfast. It's not the most significant meal of the day, it's a neutral meal, there is nothing precious. In fact, skipping breakfast won't make you fat, and breakfast won't activate your metabolism.

It's okay to avoid snacks. Eating will never help you lose weight because it does not increase your metabolism. In fact, this study shows that eating snacks contributes to obesity and fatty liver disease.

Your metabolism will not slow down. In fact, fasting boosts your metabolism and helps you maintain more muscle when you lose weight.

No need to worry, as it is not dangerous for your health. Ready? Let's start.

Now here is an example of how to follow a simple 16:8 program

Day 1, do not eat after dinner

Consuming your usual meals throughout the day, but stop eating after dinner.

You are unlikely to be really hungry between 8 p.m. and 9 p.m. after dinner at 7 p.m. But this is where you relax on the sofa, watch TV or hang out with loved ones to relax. And it's usually come with popcorn, crisps, or ice cream.

Tips to help you at night:

- Drink a cup of water or a cup of soothing herbal tea instead of eating.
- Brush your teeth. The mint flavor can help control cravings. It also sends a subliminal message saying that you have finished your meals for the day or that you should brush your teeth again. It is a sufficient barrier to prevent you from eating.
- Sleep it off. It's okay because you've been eating all day and having dinner.

Day 2, late breakfast

Hello! You just did a 12 hour fast.

Your last meal was at 7:00 p.m. last night and it is now 7:00 a.m. It's been 12 hours. You haven't eaten for half a day. You have a balanced diet and a 50:50 fasting ... 12 hours of food and 12 hours of fasting. This is a good thing.

It wasn't that hard, was it? All you are required to do was stop eating after dinner. Time flies when you sleep!

But now it's the morning race. You have to leave the house as soon as possible or you will be late. So eat as fast as you can or grab something to eat in the moving car. But why?

Delay breakfast today. Eat when it's convenient for you. Drink water, coffee, or tea instead.

There is nothing extreme about delaying the first meal of the day until it's convenient for you. Like after arriving at the office or when the kids were taken to school instead of the morning rush.

After you start working, calm down. Check your emails, check your schedule, plan your day. You don't have to have breakfast or coffee while you do all of this.

- 10 a.m. It's time to have breakfast without the chaos.
- 12 at noon. Lunch time. You are probably not hungry because you just ate. The clock says it's time for lunch, but your body doesn't. It's acceptable to wait to eat until you feel hungry again.
- 2 p.m. You are hungry now, have a good lunch.
- Dinner at 7 p.m.

Expand the above steps: do not eat after dinner, postpone breakfast until 10:00 a.m.

Day 3, do not eat a snack

Very well! You just did a 15 hour fast.

You had dinner last night at 7 p.m., stopped eating after dinner and postponed breakfast until 10 a.m. Today, after lunch, do not eat before dinner.

Tips to help you avoid snacks:

- Now you only have fews hours to dinner. You know you will eat soon. All you have to do is wait.
- Hunger comes in waves. It's temporary, it's not going to get worse over time, it's going to decrease.
- The hunger may not even be real. You might be thirsty. Maybe it's an afternoon snack habit. Maybe you are stressed, anxious, worried, sad, or bored, then you have to eat. Drink water, coffee, or tea instead.
- Keep busy. Find a job, a chore, go for a walk, or visit a friend. Before you realize it, it's time to head home for the dinner that awaits you.

Dinner at 7 p.m.

Expand the steps above: do not eat after dinner, postpone breakfast until 10:00 am, do not snack between meals.

Day 4, skip breakfast

You did it! You fasted for 15 hours and you didn't snack.

You had dinner at 7 p.m. last night, stopped eating after dinner, postponed breakfast until 10 a.m., and didn't have a snack between lunch and dinner.

Skip breakfast today while waiting another hour to eat. This makes lunch the first meal of the day at 11 a.m.

Repeat the skills you learned:

- You practiced mindful eating when you were not eating while doing some other activity.
- You didnt eat out of thirst, habit, or emotion while waiting to eat until you were really hungry.
- You have felt a short-term hunger. Do the tricks that helped you deal with the hunger waves until they disappeared.

Dinner at 7 p.m.

Expand the above steps: don't eat after dinner, skip breakfast, don't snack between lunch and dinner.

Day 5, repeat

Congratulations! You just did a 16 hour fast.

You had dinner last night at 7pm, you skipped breakfast eating your first meal at 11am, you didn't have a snack, you didn't eat again until 7pm.

This is an intermittent fasting protocol called the 16/8 Method, popularized by Martin Berkhan. It has several variations. It's popular because most of us aren't very hungry in the morning, so it's easy to skip breakfast.

Your feeding window is reduced to ⅓ of the day (8 hours). You have tipped the scales toward a greater fasting window of ⅔ of the day (16 hours). The therapeutic effects come into play.

Repeat: skip breakfast, no snacks between lunch and dinner, don't eat after dinner.

(Optional) Switch to other extended variations of intermittent fasting. Apply the principle of breaking your fast in small but easily achievable steps over a period of time and continue until you get there.

Is Intermittent Fasting Right For You?

We have already discussed this in the first chapter. Fasting, like eating a low-carb, high-fat diet, is another way to lose weight and improve your health. But the effectiveness of these tools depends on the ability to use them consistently over the long term.

Here are some benefits and drawbacks to aim your decision:

- It's simple and easy to follow because you just skip one or more meals when you're not hungry or too busy to eat.
- You can adapt it to your lifestyle, for example, organizing special occasions, holidays.
- However, there is hunger (real or not). You must develop the ability to overcome the ebb and flow of

hunger by being more aware of the reason for your eating. But since it is a skill, you can learn it.

CHAPTER THREE: EXERCISING AND EATING RIGHT FOR A HEALTHY LIFESTYLE

Nutrition is important for physical fitness. Eating a well-balanced diet can assist you in getting the calories and nutrients you need to fuel your daily activities, including regular exercise.

When it comes to eating foods to improve physical performance, it's not as easy as choosing veggies over donuts. You must consume the appropriate kinds of foods at the appropriate times of the day.

Learn about the importance of workout snacks, healthy breakfasts, and meal plans.

Start well

Your first meal of the day is significant. And regular eating breakfasts have been associated with a lower risk of obesity, heart disease and diabetes. Starting your day with a strong meal can assist you to replenish your blood sugar, which your body needs to fuel your brain and muscles.

Consuming a healthy breakfast is particularly significant on days when physical activity is the order of the day. Skipping breakfast can make you feel dizzy or feel lethargic during exercise.

Choosing the right kind of breakfast is essential. Many individual rely on simple carbohydrates to start their day. A white bagel or donut won't keep you satisfied for long.

In comparison, a breakfast rich in fiber and protein can fend off hunger pangs for a long time and provide the necessary energy to continue your exercise.

Follow these tips for a healthy breakfast:

- Instead of eating high-sugar cereals made from refined grains, try oatmeal, oat bran, or other high- fiber whole grains. Then add protein, such as milk, yogurt, or chopped nuts.
- If you are making waffles or pancakes, replace some of the flour with whole grain options. Then mix a little cottage cheese into the dough.
- If you prefer toast, choose whole grain bread. So combine it with an egg, peanut butter or some other source of protein.

Count on the right carbohydrates

Thanks to low-carb diets, carbs get a bad rap. But carbs are the body's main source of energy. About 45-65% of your total daily calories should come from carbohydrates. This is especially true if you are training.

It's important to get the appropriate kind of carbohydrate. Many people depend on the simple carbohydrates found in sweets and processed foods. Instead, you should concentrate on eating complex carbohydrates found in whole grains, fruits, vegetables and beans.

Whole grains have more resistance than refined grains because you digest them more slowly.

They can let you feel fuller for longer and fuel your body throughout the day. They can also help stabilize blood sugar. Finally, these quality grains contain the vitamins and minerals you need to keep your body functioning at its best.

Put protein in your snacks and meals

Protein is needed to help your body grow and recover. Protein is also vital for building and repairing muscle, helping you reap the benefits of your workout. It can be an energy source when carbs are scarce, but it is not the primary source of fuel during workout.

Adults is required to consume about 0.8 g of protein per day per kilogram of body weight. There is ò equivalent to about 0.36 grams of protein per kilogram of body weight. Athletes and the elderly may need even more ù .

Proteins can come from:
- Red meats like steak and lamb
- Poultry like chicken and turkey
- Fish like salmon and tuna
- Legumes such as beans and lentils
- Dairy products like milk and yogurt
- Eggs

For healthier options, choose the lean protein low in saturated fats and trans fats. Reduce the quantity of processed meat and red meat you eat.

Increase your consumption of fruits and vegetables

Vegetable and fruits are rich sources of natural fiber, vitamins, minerals, and other compounds that your body needs to function properly. In addition, they are very low in fat and calories. Make sure a laqrge part of your plate is made up of fruits and vegetables at each meal.

Try to "eat the rainbow" by selecting veggies and fruits of different colors. This will help you take advantage of the full range of vitamins, minerals and antioxidants that the manufacturing department has to offer.

Each time you go shopping, consider picking out a new fruit or vegetable to try. For snacks, keep the nuts in the gym bag and the raw vegetables in the refrigerator.

Choose healthy fats

Unsaturated fat can help reduce inflammation and provide calories. Although fat is the primary fuel in aerobic exercise, we store enough fat in the body to fuel even the longest workouts. However, the intake of healthy unsaturated fats help to provide you with the essential fatty acids and calories to keep you moving.

Healthy options include:

- seeds
- nuts
- avocados
- oils, such as olive oil
- olives

Refuel before exercise

When it comes to getting the most out of pre or post workout energy, it's important to strike the right balance between carbohydrates and protein. The pre-workout snacks that combine carbohydrates with protein can make you feel more energized than the junk foods made from simple sugars and too much fats.

Consider stocking your gym bag and fridge with some of these simple snacks:

Bananas

Bananas are very much rich in magnesium and potassium, which are important nutrients for the daily intake. Eating a banana will assist in replenishing these minerals by providing natural sugars to fuel your workout. To add protein, eat your banana with a peanut butter serving.

Berries, oranges and grapes

These fruits are all full of water, vitamins, and minerals. They're easy on your gut, provide a quick energy boost, and help keep you hydrated. Consider combining them with a serving of protein yogurt.

Nuts

Nuts are an excellent source of healthy fats for the heart and also provide protein and essential nutrients. They can offer a sustainable source of energy for your workout.

Combine them with fresh or dried fruit for a healthy dose of carbs. However, try these options to see how they work. Foods high in fat can slow digestion and cause food to stay in the stomach for a long time if training is rapid.

Nut butter

Many supermarkets sell nut butter packaging that doesn't require refrigeration and can be easily stored in a gym bag. For a tasty combination of protein and carbohydrates, you can spread peanut butter on:

- a banana
- an apple
- a slice of whole-grain bread
- whole-grain crackers

If you don't like nut butter, try almond butter, soy butter, or other high protein alternatives.

Don't cut too many calories

If you'd like to lose weight or tone your body, you might be tempted to cut a lot of calories from your meals. Cutting back on calories is a fundamental part of losing weight, but you can go too far.

Dieting should never make you feel exhausted or sick. These are signs that you are not getting the calories you need for good health and fitness.

A diet that contains 1,200 to 1,500 calories per day is suitable for most women looking to lose weight safely. A daily diet of 1,500 to 1,800 calories is suitable for most men trying to lose weight.

If you are very active or don't want to lose weight while exercising, you may need to eat more calories. Talk to your nutritionist or doctor to find out how many calories you need to maintain your lifestyle and your fitness goals.

Balance is the key

As you adopt an active lifestyle, you will likely discover which foods provide the most energy and which have the negative effects. The secret is to learn to listen to your body and find a balance between what's right for you and what's feels right.

Follow these tips:

- Try to make breakfast a part of your routine.
- Choose complex carbohydrates, the lean protein sources, healthy fats and a wide variety of fruits and vegetables.

- Fill your refrigerator and sports bag with healthy workout snacks.

The balance of carbohydrates, protein and other nutrients can help fuel your workouts.

REASONS TO EXERCISE AND EAT RIGHT APART FROM WEIGHT LOSS

If the latest ads and magazine covers are any indication, it seems like weight loss is on everyone's mind these days. And while a healthy weight is a great goal, when it comes to eating well and exercising, it shouldn't be the only goal. In fact, counting all the reasons for eating right and exercising, we don't even know if it should be in the top ten. Admit it: the number on the scale is not a reliable indicator of overall health. Worse, a study found that people who diet or exercise just to lose weight quit much sooner than individuals who make healthy changes for some other reasons. Oh, and they don't really lose weight in the long run. Researchers found that the most effective motivation for maintaining a healthy lifestyle was "feeling better about yourself" for women and "better health" for men.

And yes, both are great reasons to exercise and eat well, but these are merely a drop of water in a big ocean when we talk about all the good things you will bring into your life. Here are 44 scientific reasons to start living a healthier life today that have nothing to do with your weight.

THE BEST REASONS TO BREAK A SWEAT

1. Works like an antidepressant.

Whether you suffer from winter sadness or chronic depression, sadness can make everything in life more difficult. Antidepressant medication has been a boon to many people, but one study found that people with depression who exercise aerobically show as much improvement in symptoms as people who take medication. In fact, after five months, 60 to 70 percent of people couldn't even be classified as having depression. Better yet, a follow-up study found that the effects of exercise lasted longer than those of the drug.

2. Reduces stress and anxiety.

Exercising the body is one of the fastest ways to clear the stress hormone cortisol from your system and calm your restless mind. Plus, new study points to the fact that ice cream or other "comfort foods" don't affect stress levels much, not that we have anything against an occasional monkey ball!

3. Increase creativity.

The next time the newsroom arrives or you need some new ideas for your service meeting, try walking around the block. A recent study found that walking improves convergent and divergent thinking, both types associated with increased creativity.

4. Eliminate allergies.

Sneezing, watery eyes, etc. it can really take the fun out of a workout, but there's a good reason to buckle up your sneakers, even with an allergy attack. Researchers in Thailand have reported that running for 30 minutes can reduce sneezing, itching, stuffiness and runny nose by up to 90%.

5. Strengthen your heart.

It may appear like your heart is pounding during those uphill sprints, but your ticker will thank you for it later. Exercise minimizes the risk of heart disease and related conditions and strengthens the heart muscle. So, the next time you sweat during the spinning class, imagine it's a Valentine's Day card for your body.

6. It helps you resist temptation.

They don't call "runner's high" for nothing! Whether you are addicted to sugar, cigarettes or even heroin, exercise can play a big role in resistance to your favorite substance. In one study, scientists found that injecting endorphins released during exercise acts on the same neural pathways as addictive substances.

7. Reduces the risk of metabolic syndrome...

If there is one modern health villain, it would be scary metabolic syndrome. Composed of three factors - increased blood pressure/cholesterol, high blood sugar, and excess fat around the waist - this is one of the strongest indicators of premature death. But before you begin to plan the funeral (open bar, smoking machines, and a 12-piece band, take a look!), Researchers say exercise can almost completely eliminate metabolic syndrome and even reverse the damage. However, not all exercises work the same, as the study shows intensity is key. So instead of maintaining a steady pace, try intervals that increase and decrease your heart rate.

8. ... and it also reduces the risk of several other diseases.

Many types of heart disease, cancer, diabetes, lung disease - we would be here all day if we listed all the diseases that exercise reduces risk for. Exercise is a health prevention superstar who was recently declared "a wonderful medicine that prevents almost all diseases, is 100% effective and has few side effects". Best of all, we don't have to wait for FDA approval for this magic cure-all!

9. Protects your eyes.

We hate to say it, but you're looking at a screen right now. Welcome to the eye-strain club! But recent research has revealed that one of the best ways to protect your eyes and stave off age-related vision loss is through cardiovascular exercise. In one study, active mice retained twice as many neurons in the retina as sedentary hairballs. But that's not just a benefit for all four legs; a separate study found a similar correlation in humans.

10. Adds years to your life ...

People who exercise live longer. Yes, we said it. Study has shown that you can add up to seven years to your life by doing at least 200 minutes of exercise in a week (that's just three days of training for 50 minutes), regardless of your weight.

11. ...and life to your years.

Better yet, those extra years will be happy ones: A recent study found that people who exercise reported feeling happier, more energetic and more enthusiastic about life than their fellow TV addicts.

12. It makes you respect your body.

It is extremely easy to focus on the abdomen or bikini bridges or other (possibly inaccessible) physical attributes. But as an alternative to getting caught up in the comparisons, strap on your shoes and hit the gym. Making use of our bodies not only strengthens them, but also increases our gratitude for all the interesting things they can do, and study supports this. After all, being an sportsperson has nothing to do with the mirror - that's how your body can move.

13. Strengthen the bones.

Bone density might not be the sexiest topic, but we all need to be aware of it, especially since it helps us maintain a strong and mobile body. And according to a landmark study, the best way to increase bone density and reduce the risk of fractures and osteoporosis in older people is through strength training, such as running or dancing. Researchers found that adults who work out moderately or intensely had better bone density than those who exercised little or no exercise. Keep it up: Adults who quit exercising later in life lost bone mass, despite exercising regularly in their youth.

14. It saves money.

We know. Gym membership is expensive. Household equipment can be an investment. And have you recently reviewed any running shoes? But it turns out that investing in good shape is as frugal as it is smart. A Fortune 500 company estimates that for every dollar spent on preventive health, including exercise, $ 2.71 is saved in future health care costs. It's a smart practice to embrace as a CEO of healthcare as well.

15. Help your fertility.

Is there a child in your future? Better hit the ground with the weight. Harvard researchers discovered that men who workout had a higher concentration of sperm in their semen and the semen was of above-average quality. Women also increase fertility while running (whether with kettlebells, yoga or ...). A meta-analysis that looked at about 27,000 women found that those who exercised had lower overall infertility rates, higher implantation rates, and lower spontaneous abortion rates. One caveat: Women who exercise too much or too intensely have compromised their fertility, so it's all about balance. Researchers recommend going to the gym three times a week for an hour at a time.

16. It makes you a god or goddess of sex.

Good news for both women and men: sweating in the gym can improve the sweating in the bedroom. But in this case, women really get a score (ahem), since certain exercises have been associated with "coregasmos," or having an orgasm with abdominal work. (A strong abdomen and powerful orgasms? That's good for everyone.) But, while the hanging elevations in your legs don't surprise you, you can still benefit from the increased pelvic floor strength. And another study found that men who exercise have a lower incidence of impotence and erectile dysfunction as they experience more powerful orgasms. Additionally, these guys reported having sex more often.

17. Improve self-esteem.

Mirror, mirror on the wall (of the gym), who is the most beautiful of all? It doesn't take magic to know that training makes you look better outdoors. But scientific research shows that it also makes us feel better about ourselves. In a research review on the topic, users report greater self-esteem and less impact of negative thoughts on the body. It also increases confidence at work and in other areas of life.

18. Help you sleep like a baby (or a puppy).

Having a good night's sleep is one of the most significant things you can do for your health. A nap helps your body recover and repair damage, renew your energy, and clear your mind. But sometimes sleep doesn't come easily, usually on the nights you need it most. Exercise is like the all-natural Ambien (without the weird driving stories while sleeping). In a meta-analysis that looked at several sleep studies, it is found that individuals who exercised regularly had less incidence of insomnia and better quality of sleep. Plus, for people with insomnia, adding constant daily exercise has significantly reduced their sleepless nights.

19. It doesn't just make you appear younger, it makes you become younger.

Thanks to that sweaty glow and an advanced sense of running, people who train often look younger and healthier than their friends, and now research has found that athletes are indeed younger than their same-aged peers on a cellular level. Telomeres, the cuff at the end of DNA, start for a long time at birth and gradually get shorter with age. Until recently, I thought - that we could not make big -chose to change that, but a new study has shown that endurance athletes have more telomeres than their peers, while a second study showed that moderate exercise can lengthen telomeres by up to 10 percent. You can now feel free to lie about your age with impunity!

20. It pumps you up.

You don't necessarily need a scientist to tell you that training builds muscle and coordination. If you've ever had to lift a 50-pound bag of kitty litter from the lowest shelf in the supermarket or remove 60 inches of snow from a sidewalk, you'll be grateful for all the sweating sessions that make it a game of play. 'child. (It's just part of becoming an everyday hero.)

21. Eliminate bad fats and increase good fats. (Yes, there is good fat!)

Brown fat is a metabolic benefit, and hip and thigh fat in women has some possible hormonal benefits as well. But the only type you definitely don't want is visceral fat, the type in your belly wrapped around your internal organs, which can cause a lot of damage. Exercise to the rescue! We know that sweating can reduce fat in general, but belly fat is particularly sensitive to exercise, and a study last year found that high-intensity interval training destroyed belly fat more quickly.

22. It makes you a great example for your loved ones.

We don't want to scare you, but people are watching you. Whether your friends, your parents, your siblings, your better half (or just the lovely house nearby), your circle of friends and family, watch what you are doing and take note. And your workout encourages others to do the same. We regularly reflect the other people around us in our actions and behaviors. Therefore, know that every time you go to the gym, you are setting an example by encouraging others to do the same. And the more this is done by us, the better: when it comes to cardio, nothing is more fun than a conga line, right?

23. It makes you smarter.

So much for the silly stereotype of the bodybuilder: Building muscle also helps build brain cells. A meta-analysis of the effects of workout on the brain found that fitness improves memory, increases cognition, increases brain volume, helps you learn faster, and even makes you a better reader. Plus, recent studies have shown that training helps prevent cognitive decline with age and diseases like Alzheimer's disease.

24. Control of chronic pain.

When you live with chronic pain, getting out of bed is difficult, let alone getting out to pump some iron or run. However, research shows that a moderate exercise program offers both short and long term improvements for people with chronic pain, even if the underlying condition persists. In short, exercise may not solve all of your problems, but it will help you cope better.

THE BEST REASONS TO START HEALTHY EATING

1. Lubricate your wallet.

Oh kale, why do you have to cost so much? People often complain that healthy foods is more expensive than processed junk food. And a recent study found that whatever they produce and lean meat adds about $ 1.50 a day to food costs. But before swapping that apple for an apple pancake, the researchers went on to say that when we include the cost savings from preventing health problems - a savings of $ 2.71 for every dollar spent - you still come out way ahead.

2. It makes you more excited.

An apple a single day keeps the blues away, say New Zealand researchers. The study found that on days when young adults ate more fruits and vegetables, they felt calmer, happier and more energetic than normal. And scientists say it wasn't just happy people who ate the most honey. The data showed that these positive feelings were a direct result of the salad.

3. Protect your bones.

No walkers for you! A healthy diet that is very rich in vitamin D, calcium, and folic acid supports your skeleton, preventing osteoporosis and fractures in the elderly.

4. Increase your fertility.

It's for expectant parents: A recent study found that eating swimmers (like fish) stimulate your swimmers (like sperm). For ladies, the effect of a good diet is even more powerful, because another study revealed that access to a wide variety of healthy foods was the number one predictor of high fertility rates among women who don't use birth control.

5. Get over the cramps.

The fibers of fruits and vegetables fight bloating, magnesium-rich foods (like chocolate!) Prevent cramps, iron it in red meat helps the fatigue, the calcium in dairy products is soothing and zinc in plants green helps to ease mood swings.

6. Provides a foolproof immune system.

In life, you will share pens, exchange business cards, and greet people of questionable hygiene. Translation: you will be affected by germs. But research has shown that eating fruits and vegetables five times a day can boost your immune system and prevent five (or more) days of illness. One research found that individuals who ate more produce fell ill less often, regardless of what other foods they ate. Another argument that carrots and crackers can coexist. And you might want to season these veggies with garlic - people who ate cloves every day had 64% fewer colds and recovered faster than those who had less smelly breath.

7. Corrects your DNA.

Have you ever complained about your "bad DNA" which, for example, gave you a car horn or a family history of a heart attack? Well, don't complain anymore. A recent study in the new field of epigenesis found that a healthy diet can "turn on" good DNA and "turn off" bad DNA, leading to long term and even generational benefits. So while you probably can't get a nutritious nose job, you can eat your way to reduce heart disease and spare your children the inheritance of risk.

8. It can help treat irritable bowel syndrome (IBS).

IBS is to stomach aches what Godzilla is to the Geico gecko. Patients experience debilitating pain, swelling, persistent constipation, and embarrassing (sometimes public) manifestations of diarrhea. But new study has found a link between the bacteria that live in a person's instinct and their possibility of having IBS, saying that consuming probiotics has helped most patients find a truce. And don't just go looking for yogurt to get your fix.

9. Make your (future) children smarter ...

There is nothing strange about this: A pediatric study shows that pregnant women who eat a diet high in omega-3 fatty acids, especially DHA, continue to have children with a higher IQ at age four than mothers who avoid seafood. And another study presented that children who took DHA supplements or ate a lot of fish also had cognitive improvements.

10. ... And it also makes you smarter.

Fish oil isn't just for kids! Eating more fish can increase your cognition. But it's not only a matter of pulling the (fishing) line; a diet rich in healthy fats, protein-producing and antioxidants increases cognition and still prevents more memory loss ù more later in life, says a neuroscientist study.

11. It is the best workout intensifier.

Just as exercise can help you eat better, eating better can help you crash at the gym. Exercise, by definition, breaks you down. It's hard on the muscles, bones, and cardiovascular system. It is how your body heals all the damage that makes you stronger and healthy food support that growth and recovery process. Good carbohydrates enhance your endurance, protein builds and maintains muscle, and minerals and vitamins keep everything working together as it should.

12. It gives you chills.

Tryptophan can help you relax. Researchers found that men without tryptophan experienced an immediate increase in anxiety and some even had panic attacks. But once they got the tryptophan again, they calmed down like babies in a bubble bath. And there's no need to remove the turkey stick - tryptophan is found in many healthy foods, such as dark chocolate, oats, nuts, seeds, eggs, fish, and dairy products.

13. Provides clearer skin.

Breakouts in high school are expected with fluctuating hormones in teens. But, unfortunately, adulthood does not guarantee the end of the acne era. If you're still struggling with red spots, take a look at your plate. Scientists say you can eat to lighten your skin. Sugary foods, dairy products, processed grains have all been associated with outbreaks of rosacea and acne. And new research has shown that eliminating these foods seems to solve the problem. While the effects aren't consistent across the board, the American Academy of Dermatology says it's worth trying to rule out these things and see if it helps.

14. Your sexual desire is amplified.

Although many foods (like wine, chocolate, and oysters) have been hailed as aphrodisiacs, in scientific studies the effects have been attributed primarily to the placebo effect. But new data suggests we're looking at the spice corridor. Researchers found that eating healthy spices such as saffron and ginger significantly improved sexual desire and performance in both sexes. Stay away from alcohol, however. While "liquid courage" can improve your flirting game, researchers have found that it significantly improves desire and significantly reduces performance.

15. Prevents insomnia.

With around 50% of adults experiencing at least one insomnia outbreak that lasts longer than three weeks, insomnia is one of the top complaints people have about their health. Fortunately, good nutrition can help you get your zzz back. One study showed that adults who drank a delicious sour cherry smoothie got an average of 90 minutes extra sleep per night. Other study has shown that magnesium, found in foods such as dark chocolate and whole oats, helps people fall asleep faster with fewer episodes of waking up at night. Finally, in a third research, individuals who ate fermented dairy products, like yogurt and kefir, slept more and slept better.

16. Soothes sore muscles.

According to multiple studies, what you eat can greatly affect the speed and ability of your muscles to recover after a workout. (Eat right and you will be able to sit like a normal person after squats in the bootcamp.) The most important factor, according to research, was getting enough protein, as this nutrient is responsible for building and repairing skeletal muscles, but blueberries also offered measurable relief.

17. It gives you more energy.

The next time you feel exhausted, ditch the "energy" drinks and go to the blender. Long-term caffeine abuse can not only exhaust you by ruining your sleep, but it can also exacerbate the effects of stress, which also makes you mentally fatigued. Instead, whip up a smoothie with balanced carbohydrates for a quick energy and protein complex to improve performance and aid recovery. A study of athletes showed that those who drank the protein shake showed a significant improvement in their performance in an athletic test compared to those who relied only on carbohydrates.

18. Reduces the need for bad food.

Classify it in something odd, but true: Eating a salmon omelet can ward off Swedish seafood cravings. Researchers discovered that starting the day with a high protein meal for breakfast helped reduce cravings for junk food throughout the day. Instead of feeling deprived of their favorite treats, subjects reported not thinking too much about the treats. Researchers believe that eating a healthy breakfast with high protein content increases dopamine levels in the brain. Since 91% of us report having intense cravings for food, according to a Tufts study, we'll see you at the breakfast bar.

19. Makes you a faster runner.

The turtles that finally try to beat the hares shouldn't look past their plate, the researchers say. In one study, runners who ate beets saw a significant increase in their endurance and speed. But prefer whole beets to beet juice or extracts, as the effect was more pronounced when consuming the food. Another research found that individuals who ate a Mediterranean-style diet (high in fish, olive oil and nuts, and light in ice cream) increased their resistance to running, increased their exercise tolerance and exhibited improvements in their cardiovascular health.

20. It will save you money in life.

Taking good care of your health will bring you not only all the benefits we have listed and many more, but also confidence and self-awareness in all aspects of your life, so enjoy your meal!

CHAPTER FOUR: TYPES OF INTERMITTENT FASTING

There are different ways to perform intermittent fasting, and that's awesome. If this is something that interests you, you can find the type that will work best for your lifestyle, which will increase your chances of success.

5:2 INTERMITTENT FASTING AKA. THE FAST DIET

How: 2 days a week, limit calories to 500-600, 5 days a week, eat normally.

It is among the most common intermittent fasting methods. The idea is to eat as usual for five days (not counting calories) and then the other two eat 500 or 600 calories per day respectively for women and men. Fasting days are days of your choice.

The idea is that short periods of fasting will keep you obedient; if you are hungry while on your fast day, you just have to wait until tomorrow, when you can "party" again. "Some people say, 'I can do it all for two days, but it's too much to cut what I eat for the seven days. "For these individuals, a 5: 2 approach may work for them when it comes to reducing calories during the week.

That said, we don't recommend fasting on days when you can do a lot of resistance exercise. If you are getting ready for a bike ride or a jog (or if you run for weeks with lots of miles), ask yourself if this type of fasting can work with your workout schedule or talk to a sports nutritionist.

Who is the approach for?

Although intermittent fasting is very safe for people in good health and well-fed, it is not actually suitable for the whole world.

Some people should avoid dietary restrictions and fasting. These include:

- People with a history of eating disorders.
- People who experience frequent drops in blood sugar.
- Pregnant women, nursing mothers, adolescents, children and people with type 1 diabetes.
- People who are known for malnutrition, underweight or nutritional deficiencies.
- Women who are trying to conceive or who have fertility problems.

Additionally, intermittent fasting may not be as beneficial for some women as it is for men.

Some women have reported that their periods stopped by following this type of diet. However, things returned to normal when they returned to a normal diet.

Therefore, women should exercise caution when initiating any form of intermittent fasting and stop it immediately if any side effects occur.

More on the 5:2 schedule will be discussed in chapter 6.

INTERMITTENT FASTING 16/8

How: Fast for 16 hours and eat 8 hours

As a result of this 16/8 intermittent fasting schedule, you fast for 16 hours and limit your food to an 8-hour window.

It is up to you to know which 16 hours per day you decide to limit your food intake. You can choose to have a window to eat from 8 a.m. to 4 p.m., from 10 a.m. to 6 p.m., noon to 8 p.m. or any other time, as long as it is 4 p.m. without eating continuously.

Most people who take this program choose to skip breakfast instead of dinner, but different people have different rhythms of life.

The great thing is that in 16 hours you will probably be sleeping at least 7-8 hours, so we're only talking about 9-8 hours of fasting per day.

Who is the approach for?

The Fast LeanGains is for athletes and any serious weight lifter. It is not recommended for casual or novice users due to its complex planning.

Rules

- The diet should be high in protein
- You must include training while fasting (fasted training)
- You should be riding a carbohydrate bike (training days should be high in carbohydrates, while rest days should be lower in carbohydrates).
- Eating windows should be consistent.

- On workout days, your post-workout meal should be your biggest meal.
- On non-workout days, your first meal should be your biggest meal.
- Be sure to take BCAAs (Branched Chain Amino Acids) before exercising to ensure you don't lose muscle while training on an empty stomach.

Instructions

- Determine your 16 hour fasting period. Ideally, you would like the fast to last all night while you sleep. If you fast for 16 hours while you are awake, that means the 8-hour feeding window is occurring while you are asleep. For example, let's say your last meal is at 6 p.m. on Tuesday, then you fast until 10 a.m. on Wednesday. Its feeding window would be from 10:00 a.m. to 6:00 p.m.
- After deciding on the fasting period, your feeding window will be for the remaining 8 hours of the day.
- Set a time for training. Ideally, your workout window should be right before the eating window, so that your first meal of the day is the same as your post-workout meal.

What you should not do

- Don't schedule your fasting period so that your feeding window is the same time you normally sleep.

- Remember to take your BCAAs before you start your fasted training. Most protein supplements contain BCAAs.

THE 24-HOUR FAST (24 HOURS FAST ONCE A WEEK)

How: Fast 24 hours, once or twice a week

Popularized by author of Eat Stop Eat, Brad Pilon, the fast of 24 hours is a fast that lasts a whole day. You will only fast one day per week and for the other 6 days you will eat normally. The fasting for 24 hours shows a fat loss weekly. For example, if you normally eat 2,000 calories per day, that gives you a total of 14,000 calories per week. Now if you subtract one day, you've dropped to 12,000 calories.

Who is this approach for?

The 24 hours fast works great for beginners and those on occasional diets. It is the simplest of all the programs because there is only one rule to follow. People unfamiliar with intermittent fasting should start with 24 fast and, if desired, move on to other intermittent fasting programs.

Rules

- Do not eat for 24 hours

Instructions

- Choose a day you want to fast
- Set the quick start time, for example, if you decide your last meal should be at 8 p.m. on Wednesday, instead of fasting until 8 p.m. on Thursday.
- Ensure to be productive on your fast day and get your job done.

What you should not do

- Do not compensate by eating more in the other 6 days. If you start to eat more, know that you have room for cushion. For example, if you ate 400 more calories on Friday, know that you still have a deficit of 1,600 (2,000 to 400), so don't worry.
- Don't think about food while fasting. Keep your mind busy.

20/4 INTERMITTENT FASTING A.K.A. WARRIOR DIET

How: fast for 20 hours and eat for 4 hours

The Warrior's Diet is a 20-hour fasting period followed by a 4-hour feeding window. Like Leangains, the warrior's diet is also daily. The Warriors Diet was created by Ori Hofmekler and is inspired by the eating habits of Greek and Spartan warriors. With this plan, you will fast or eat small amounts of food for 18 to 20 hours. Thus, you would consume most of your daily calorie intake for the remaining 4-6 hours. Ideally, you should place the feeding window at the end of the day, as it is more convenient for after-work training sessions and family dinners. The only problem with the Warrior's Diet is that it can be difficult to try and fit your daily calorie intake with a meal. In summary, the warrior's diet consists mainly of a 20 hour fast followed by a heavy meal.

Who is this approach for?

The Warrior Diet is for people looking for an entry point for fasting. This diet is not as rigid as Leangains and it is very flexible. This diet is a favorite for individuals who like to indulge in high-calorie foods (e.g., Pizza, burgers, cakes, etc.) The Warrior's Diet is an excellent quick introductory diet. Makes the transition to traditional fasting easier as it allows you to make small snacks throughout the day as your snacks should consist of fruits and vegetables. If you want to experience fasting or get a feel for what fasting is, start with the Warrior's Diet.

Rules

- Fast for at least 18 to 20 hours.
- Snacks are limited to fruits and vegetables, sometimes a protein shake
- Maintain your protein diet (remember at least 1 gram per pound of body weight)
- Try to meet your daily calorie needs with a meal, which means you can enjoy high-calorie foods to reach your goal. Okay, technically it's not a meal, since you have 4 hours to eat whatever you want, but let's be candid, how many people still feel hungry after the first meal?

Instructions

- Determine which meal you want to put in your food window (i.e., breakfast, lunch, dinner)
- Determine the size you want the feeding window to be 4 to 6 hours, the minimum and the maximum. Your fasting period will correspond to the remaining hours of the day.
- Decide if you want to snack or end a fast during the day. Remember that your snacks should be fruit or veg and maybe a protein shake.

What you should not do

- Don't eat anything high in calories for snacks like chips, candies, pies. Only vegetables and fruits are allowed (baby carrots, spinach rolls, grapes, apples, etc.).
- Don't eat large meals outside of your eating window
- Don't constantly turn on your big meal (i.e., go from dinner one day to breakfast the next), keep it consistent.

THE 36/12 HOURS FAST (ALTERNATE DAY FAST)

How: Fast for 36 hours and eat for 12 hours

In this program, you eat every day. Basically, you eat in a 12 hour window, say 7 a.m. to 7 p.m. on Monday. Then you fast for the rest of Monday and all Tuesday. On Wednesday we eat again from 7:00 a.m. to 7:00 p.m. Rinse and repeat. During the feeding window, you can eat whatever you wish, however, it is recommended that the diet consists primarily of nutritious foods.

Who is this approach for?

The alternating diet is suitable for the general public, that is, those who follow an occasional diet. It is easy to take and apply. I would recommend this intermittent fasting program for beginners as it is not very rigid and must not be used in conjunction with a training program.

Rules

- Fast for 36 hours.
- Eat normally during the 12-hour eating window
- You can eat whatever you want, high-calorie foods in moderation, of course (unless you're seriously behind on calories and need an excess).

Instructions

- Fix the time for your 12-hour feeding window. Note that most people choose the start time as the first time they get up.
- Your fasting period will include the remaining 12 hours from that day plus the next day. You will eat the day after your fasting day.

23/1 INTERMITTENT FASTING AKA ONE MEAL A DAY

How: Fast 23 hours and eat once a day

Another popular fasting program is called one meal a day (OMAD). This is precisely the way it sounds: Pick a time of day that works for you and the only meal of the day.

I know what you're thinking - aren't you almost starving? And yes, you are right: the OMAD diet should not be done without thinking about how to get at least 1200 calories during this meal.

So if you choose this 23/1 fast, make sure your meal is filling and nutritious if you want to try OMAD.

CIRCADIAN RHYTHM FASTING

How: Begin fasting when the sun goes down and eating when the sun rises

You may have heard that our bodies were designed to follow the circadian rhythm, an internal clock that works 24/7 and regulates our energy levels according to the rhythm of the day and night.

So if you are keeping up with the rapid circadian rhythm, let daylight decide your schedule.

As soon as the sun rises, open the window to eat. As soon as it falls and it gets dark, you should start fasting.

The only downside is that success really depends on where you areliving. In some areas on our planet Earth like northern Norway, the sun never always sets 76 days a year ... and it's a fasting period that I certainly wouldn't recommend.

PROLONGED A.K.A EXTENDED FASTING

How: Fasting more than 24 hours in a month

As mentioned above, an extended or prolonged fast usually means between 24 and 96 hours of fasting. It is not recommended to do this more than once a month, and anything exceeding 48 to 72 hours of fasting should be done under the supervision of a doctor.

Yes, there are a lot of people who do not follow this recommendation and nothing happen to them but it is risky and we do not recommend it if you do not have experience faster and especially if you have one of the medical conditions described above.

CHAPTER FIVE: INTERMITTENT FASTING FOR WEIGHT LOSS

There are many ways to lose weight. The one that has become popular in recent years is the intermittent fasting.

As earlier explained, it is a form of eating that involves regular short-term fasting. Fasting for short periods of time helps people eat fewer calories and also helps optimize certain hormones related to weight control.

As long as you have not compensated by eating a lot more during the non-fasting times, these methods will lead to minimized calorie intake and help you lose belly fat and weight.

HOW DOES INTERMITTENT FASTING AFFECT YOUR HORMONES?

Body fat is the body's means of storing energy (calories). When we don't eat, the body changes a lot of things to make the stored energy more accessible.

It has to do with some changes in the activity of the nervous system, as well as a some change in several vital hormones.

Here are part of the things that change in our metabolism when we fast:

- **Insulin:** Insulin rises when we eat. When we fast, insulin drops dramatically. Lower insulin levels enable us to burn fat easier.

- **Human Growth Hormone (HGH):** Growth hormone levels can skyrocket during a fast, increasing up to 5 times. Growth hormone is a hormone that can, among other things, contribute to fat loss and muscle gain.
- **Norepinephrine (noradrenaline):** The nervous system sends norepinephrine in fat cells, which causes them to break down the fat body into free fatty acids that can be burned to produce energy.

Interestingly, despite what the advocates of 5-6 meals a day would have you believe, short-term fasting can actually increase fat burning.

Fasting for about 48 hours, the metabolism increases from 3.6 to 14 percent. However, longer periods of fasting can suppress metabolism.

INTERMITTENT FASTING HELPS YOU LOSE WEIGHT AND REDUCE CALORIES

The major reason that intermittent fasting works for weight loss is that it helps you eat fewer calories.

All of the different protocols include skipping meals during fasting times. Unless you compensate by eating a lot more during feeding times, you will be consuming fewer calories.

Intermittent fasting may result in substantial weight loss. In one review, intermittent fasting reduced body weight by 3-8% over a 3-24 week period.

When examining the rate of weight loss, individuals lost about 0.55 pounds (0.25 kg) within week with intermittent fasting, but 1.65 pounds (0.75 kg) per week with fasting every other day.

People have also lost 4-7% of their waistline, which indicates that they have lost abdominal fat. These results are very inspiring and show that intermittent fasting can be a useful aid in losing weight.

That said, the benefits of intermittent fasting go far beyond just losing weight. It also has several metabolic health benefits and may even help prevent chronic disease and increase life expectancy.

While calorie counting is not usually necessary during intermittent fasting, weight loss is primarily mediated by an overall reduction in calorie intake.

Studies comparing continuous calorie restriction and intermittent fasting show no change in weight loss if calories are combined between groups.

HOW EXACTLY DOES INTERMITTENT FASTING WORK FOR WEIGHT LOSS?

Intermittent fasting all depends on when you eat. Depending on the intermittent fasting approach, you are either reducing your eating window every day, or engaging in about 24-hour fasts once or several times a week. "One of the most widely-used intermittent fsting programs is the 16: 8 method, which involves fasting for an eight-hour window, for example, from 8 pm to 12 noon the next day.

Essentially, by limiting your food intake to a shorter window of time, you naturally decrease your calorie intake and as a result you can lose weight. (Remember that weight loss, at the most basic level, happens when you consume fewer calories than you consume each day). You are not only taking in fewer calories, but you are also slowing down your pumping which can increase fat burning.

HOW LONG WILL IT TAKE TO START LOSING WEIGHT DURING INTERMITTENT FASTING?

There are many factors that can contribute to the time it takes for the weight to start to drop. The rate of weight loss varies widely from person to person, depending on several factors including initial weight, the intermittent fasting approach used, the type (and amount) of food eaten during power windows, etc.

If you end up immediately reducing your overall calorie intake and consistently eating fewer calories than you consume, you should start losing weight immediately. However, you probably won't notice any weight loss results for at least a few weeks, adding that some early weight loss is likely due to water weight.

Depending on the number of calories you have consumed during intermittent fasting, you may see a loss in weight of around 1 to 2 pounds per week, which means that it may take eight to 10 weeks for you to notice a significant loss of weight.

Should you lose more? It could be a red flag. If you lose much weight in the first few weeks after going on an intermittent fasting program, you should probably re-evaluate your calorie intake to make sure you're getting the right nutrition to meet your body's needs.

REASONS YOU ARE NOT LOSING WEIGHT WHILE DOING INTERMITTENT FASTING

There could be several reasons. Here are 12 intermittent fasting mistakes you can make and how to fix them.

1. You eat too much during the feeding window.

As mentioned, in general, weight loss basically comes down to calories consumed versus calories lost. "If we end up consuming the same number of calories (or even more) during our feeding windows as we did before we started intermittent fasting, we won't lose weight." In other words, if we put all the calories we normally eat in the diet window, we are not really changing our diet.

How to solve this problem: try a calorie counting app. While I don't generally recommend calorie counting, it can be helpful to monitor your calorie intake for a few days using a calorie tracker app. "These apps usually tell you the approximate amount of daily calories you need to lose weight. While these estimates are often wrong, they can be used as a good starting point." The app can also reveal specific meals or foods with more calories than expected, and you can regulate your diet accordingly.

2. You are not consuming sufficient calories on non-fasting days.

When you do not consume a sufficient amount of calories a day without fasting, your body can conserve energy that you consume instead of burn.

How to solve this problem: Make a meal plan for yourself on days without fasting. "Prepare a meal plan suitable for periods without fasting that includes balanced meals with at least 300 to 500 calories per meal." Through this, you take the guesswork out of it and you can be sure that you are not saving calories for yourself.

3. You eat less nutritious foods.

While the goal of intermittent fasting is not what you eat but when you eat, that doesn't imply you can eat anything you want during feeding windows and continue to lose weight. If your diet consists mostly of high-calorie foods, such as fast food, you are unlikely to lose weight.

How to solve this problem: Focus on consuming nutrient-dense foods. Eating foods rich in lean protein, healthy fats and fiber-rich carbs will help fill you up and naturally reduce your overall calorie consumption. Do not worry, you may still enjoy your less healthy favorites like pizza and ice cream in moderation.

4. You are not fasting enough.

If you decide to take a time-limited diet approach and shorten the feeding window to just an hour or more per day, it is rare to see much more weight loss. You just aren't changing your normal eating routine enough, to be honest.

How to solve this problem: Most women are successful with a feeding window of around 10 hours, or a 14 hour fast. You can always start with a longer flow window and work your way down if the usual flow window is much longer than that.

5. You skip meals during the feeding period.

Skipping meals and not eating enough during feeding windows can make you very hungry during fasting times, increasing the likelihood that you will end up breaking your fast. Restricting yourself excessively during a feeding window can also lead to binge eating and overeating during the next feeding window, which can also increase your overall calorie intake.

How to solve this issue: Ensure you eat until you are satisfied, but not too much, during the meal windows. Martin also suggests making weekend food for the following week to make sure you don't skip meals when you're busy or miss your schedule.

6. You have chosen the wrong type of fasting plan.

There are different intermittent fasting plans. Not all plans may suit your lifestyle or help you increase your specific metabolic rate. For instance, if you are getting ready for a resistance challenge and have chosen a plan that stops you from eating in the morning when you need fuel to work out, you may fall off the intermittent fasting movement in the process (and also affect your body and performance).

How to solve this issue: Consider opting for an intermittent fasting plan that best suits your lifestyle and can be sustained over a long period of time. You can consult a licensed nutritionist to help you make this decision and assess your lifestyle and dietary needs.

7. You are not getting enough sleep.

Few studies have found a direct correlation with sleep and weight loss while following an intermittent fasting schedule; however, in general, more studies have shown a link between adequate sleep and positive weight loss results.

How to solve this problem: You have heard of it before, but make an effort to sleep at least seven hours a night. (Difficult, but do your best!)

8. You're working out too hard.

Often times, people start a new diet, such as a fasting diet, exactly the same time they decide to start a new exercise program or update the exercise program they are following. Excessive or very strenuous exercise, especially when trying to reduce your food intake, can lower energy levels and trigger hunger. Due to this fact, you can end up consuming more calories during power windows than you burn, even with strenuous exercise.

How to solve this problem: If you do all-day fasting (like the 5: 2 method, for example), be sure to do light exercise on fasting days. In general, make sure your exercise program is stimulating, but achievable and enjoyable. If you are hungry on the days you exercise, it may mean you are trying too hard.

9. You are not hydrated enough.

Not drinking enough water while fasting can not only dehydrate you, but by not drinking enough you also lose the benefits of water when it comes to starving you.

How to solve this problem: Drink more! And you can have fun with your water. Drinks approved for intermittent fasting include: hot tea, black coffee, sparkling water, iced tea, stevia tea or coffee.

10. You are not following your plan as directed.

Following an intermittent fasting diet can be difficult for some dieters because they are not used to going for long periods without eating. So if you keep cheating on your plan week after week or cutting costs, it probably isn't going to produce the weight loss benefits you expected. Therefore, you may want to reconsider if the intermittent fasting is appropriate for you and your lifestyle.

How to solve this problem: Choose an intermittent fasting plan that best suits your lifestyle and can be followed for long periods.

11. You fail to plan ahead.

Planning ahead is a significant aspect of maintaining any kind of healthy intervention.

How to solve this problem: Try to plan all your meals and snacks at least a day in advance. Have an idea of what you will prepare, including packing meals and snacks ahead of time, or reading restaurant menus to decide what to order.

12. You feel guilty because you have broken a fast.

Intermittent fasting takes practice and patience. Most people who try the intermittent fasting, whatever the method is chosen, eventually break the fast before the calendar at one time or another. If you really want to continue the fast, it's important not to feel guilty, embarrassed, or angry at yourself to do so and get back to a regular schedule as quickly as possible.

How to solve this issue: It is significant to give yourself a little grace and move on! Always remember that intermittent fasting takes a bit of trial and error, it is inevitable that your intermittent fasting schedule does not always go as planned.

HOW TO SUCCEED WITH INTERMITTENT FASTING PROTOCOL

Intermittent fasting is not necessarily easy at first, but there are hacks to make it a less difficult transition process.

Choose the best window for you: Not everyone in the world with a 16: 8 schedule has to start at the same time. So, if you're an individual who goes to bed early, early to wake up, consider starting your fast at 6:30 p.m. or 7:00 p.m. and ending it 16 hours later. The exact time you choose to have a feeding window doesn't matter as much as the length of your fasting window because cellular changes occur when the system is in digestive rest.

Start slow: If the idea of a 16 hour fast is scary, start slowly, with 12 or 13 hours. So every day try to take things a little further.

Drink plenty of water: This is especially important upon waking up in the morning, as most of us wake up dehydrated. Your hunger signal is the same as your thirst signal, so if you drink a lot of water when after waking up, your body won't think you need to eat. Take steps to stay hydrated throughout the morning, drinking water, sparkling water, regular coffee, and tea. Aim for the half of your body weight in ounces per day (for example: if you weigh 100 pounds (45 kilograms), shoot for 50 ounces (1.4 liters) of water per day). Drinking plenty of water will help prevent headaches and other detoxifying effects.

Stay busy: Most of us snack when we are bored. Avoid the desire to break your fast too soon by practicing physical activities, exercising, working hard and practicing a pass - time. And be careful when watching TV at night, if it's a noble snack, it's time for you! You may need to do something else during these hours to keep you busy, like working on the computer or pursuing that hobby that you didn't have in the morning.

Don't overthink it: Since many people are immediately intimidated into not eating for 16 hours, it can help to think outside the box. Intermittent fasting is an eating schedule, not diet, knowing that much of the challenge is mental because people assume they can't go that long without eating. I believe the 16: 8 protocol is better because it is not as extreme as some of the other forms, so most people can maintain the fasting lifestyle for the long term.

Stay positive: Do not fast so much that you are afraid, because then it becomes negative and is no longer very useful and unsustainable. Food must be enjoyed and provide us with many necessary nutrients. The moment he becomes the enemy, we have to rethink what we do and why we feel it.

There's an app for that - if the technology helps you stay focused and honest, download a quick tracker app. I prefer the **Life Fasting Tracker**, which also allows friends to participate in circles to find out who is fasting and when. Plus, using an app to track what you're eating is a good way to make sure you're getting enough of the right things. **MyFitnessPal** is a particularly useful tool to aid in the process of nutrient monitoring.

Join a group: Many of us need the crowd that goes with doing the group things. You can gather like-minded friends informally through a Facebook group, or you can try using a certified coach. Groups are a best way to lose weight, as they provide the necessary support and encouragement throughout the fasting process, in addition to being a great place to exchange recipes and ideas and solve problems, if needed.

Plan Ahead: As with most common "diets," planning ahead is the key to success with intermittent fasting. After all, you only have a few hours to get your nutrients. Getting enough calories during the feeding window is also very important, as insufficient nutrition can adversely affect your hormonal health, knowing that planning meals and snacks in advance will help you get enough food. integers during the power window. A great means to do this is to add snacks and eat every two to three hours. Some are successful by eating three meals spaced apart, while others eat two and snack between them.

Keep healthy meals: Eating lots of junk food during the eight-hour window won't help you lose weight. There will be results that you will only see with fasting, as this usually reduces the total number of foods and calories consumed. However, if the food is very high in calories and not very healthy during the period of consumption, this may negate the goal. There may still be health benefits of fasting, but we still don't know for sure from the current research we have.

CHAPTER SIX: THE 5:2 METHOD STEP BY STEP

Fasting for two days in a week can come back and bite you. The 5:2 diet, a kind of intermittent fasting popularized by British presenter Michael Mosley and late-night presenter Jimmy Kimmel. Advocates showed it can reduce the risk of chronic disease and promote weight loss. Additionally, some studies have linked the fasting schedule to longevity. While the 5: 2 fast diet may work for some people, it certainly isn't for everyone. Here's what you must know before joining this diet trend.

WHAT IS THE 5:2 FAST DIET?

The 5:2 fast diet is a form of fasting in which partakers eat about 25% of their recommended calorie required (about 500-600 calories) during two scheduled fasting days, then eat normally the other five days of the week. People often alternate their fasting days (like scheduling them on Mondays and Thursdays) so they aren't one after the other.

Many followers take the 5:2 diet to the extreme, consuming zero calories on fasting days. Others place restrictions on fasting free days after a high fat ketogenic diet. You may also be aware of the 4: 3 diet, which is the same concept, but you should fast for three days instead of two.

CAN THE 5:2 FAST DIET HELP YOU LOSE WEIGHT?

It really depends on the circumstances. The theory is that intermittent fasting limits your eating options, and you'll lose weight just by eating fewer calories overall. This is because many of us eat according to the scenario, not according to the level of hunger. For example, if you fast in a Tuesday meeting, which always includes fresh donuts, it may prevent you from eating more caloric foods than you would eat. However, you could probably achieve the same goal by eating a healthy snack about 30 minutes before the meeting and skipping fried, mushy treats just because you've already eaten something more nutritious.

If you have a general calorie deficit during the week, then yes, you will probably lose weight. But this diet only controls calorie intake two days a week; During the remaining five days of the week, you have the option to eat almost anything you want; Therefore, in the grand scheme of things, your calorie intake may not be drastically reduced at the end of the week to warrant weight loss.

IS THE 5:2 FAST DIET GOOD FOR YOUR HEALTH?

Remember, there is no one-size-fits-all approach to food and nutrition. The first red flag for me when I look at the 5: 2 diet is that 500 calories is not sufficient food to support even basic bodily functions while at rest (translation: you would practically pass out eating those few calories a day, especially repeatedly overtime). You must also be careful with exercise on low calorie days, as you probably won't have enough fuel to fuel your workout. In addition, there is not enough food to meet the daily needs of important vitamins and minerals; if you choose to try the 5: 2 diet, you'll want to at least start taking a multivitamin on fasting days to make up for the lack of nutrients you're getting from food.

When it comes to fasting days, going for a long time without eating can also set you up for overeating, creating a difficult cycle to break as long-term fasting can interfere with your body's hunger signals and metabolism. Restriction can also build an unhealthy relationship with food, which is why this diet is not particularly recommended for people with active eating disorders or with a history of eating disorders. This diet is also not suitable for women who are trying to conceive, pregnant, or breastfeeding. If you have a history of hypoglycemia, diabetes, or nutritional deficiencies, the 5: 2 diet is not recommended.

If you're still intrigued by the diet and think it might work for you, my biggest tip is to limit yourself to nutrient- dense foods that provide more bulk on fast days. For example, a standard Dunkin Donuts muffin contains over 500 calories; don't waste calories one day all with just a muffin, please! Prioritize foods like fruits and vegetables which are high in fiber and contain a large number of minerals and vitamins, as well as soups which are volume based and can fill you up with fewer calories. Choose the protein sources lean that are not fried or greasy, and also make sure to stay hydrated throughout the day. The last thing you want is burning your fasting few calories on soda or fruit juice.

IS THE 5:2 DIET SUSTAINABLE FOR LONG-TERM WEIGHT LOSS?

There is very little study on the 5: 2 diet period, and even less over an extended period. A gradual and moderate reduction in calories, along with maintaining hydration and choosing foods that are higher in nutrients, can lead to long-lasting and lasting weight loss over time. The 5: 2 diet has very extreme calorie fluctuations throughout the week. I would say a more modest but sustainable daily calorie reduction where you can still incorporate your favorite foods and not starve. It reminds me of the expression Hara Hachi bu, a Confucian saying recited before every meal in the community of Okinawa, Japan (which is considered a " blue zone " and is home to the world's oldest women). The phrase prompts Okinawans to desist from eating when they are 80% full and helps to avoid overeating. Eating carefully, staying hydrated, and planning ahead are your best secrets to successful long-term weight loss/management.

WHAT YOU CAN AND CANNOT EAT ON THE 5: 2 FAST DIET

Here are some strict rules about what you can and cannot eat on the 5: 2 Fast Diet.

Authorized foods:

There are no fast and hard instructions about what to eat on the 5: 2 diet, so you may eat anything you want on fast days, as long as you're within the calorie limits. Usually, people eat low calorie foods on fasting days. This can include vegetables, fish, soup, eggs, and lean meat, as well as non-calorie drinks such as water and coffee or black tea. You can eat up to three times within a day on a fasting day. Since there is no official 5: 2 diet list or 5: 2 diet recipes, you just have to control your calorie intake, instead of macronutrients and the like. Here are some examples of foods you can eat on 5: 2 diets:

- Fresh fruits
- Fresh vegetables
- Lean meats and poultry
- Low-fat dairy
- Fish and seafood
- Whole grains
- Healthy fats (for example avocados, olive oil, coconut oil, flaxseed oil, and nuts)
- Legumes (such as beans and lentils)
- Nuts and seeds
- Limited amounts of sugar, honey, and sweet treats.

Food not allowed

With a 500-600 calorie limit on fasting days with the 5: 2 diet, you really need to be wise about what foods you eat. This is why the GI becomes particularly important. Stick to foods and drinks that are high in protein and have a low GI index. You will feel more ù pi complete ù long and you will not feel the feared collapse of sugar and an empty stomach feeling.

Some foods and drinks to avoid on fasting days include:

Typical high carbohydrate foods, such as pasta, pizza, white rice, and bread: High carbohydrate foods are not only full of empty calories, but also have a high GI, which means they wreak havoc on the blood sugar levels. Sudden fluctuations in blood sugar make fasting much more difficult and negate the benefits of fasting, like increased insulin sensitivity and fat loss.

Anything that contains refined or processed sugars (high fructose corn syrup, table sugar, agave nectar, and so on): As you try to avoid meeting your calorie limits in fasts days with empty calories, you shouldn't waste those 500 or 600 calories on simple sugars.

Honey and maple syrup, two sweeteners that are generally better choices to satisfy your sweet tooth (but always in moderation), should also be eliminated on the two days of the week that you are fasting. If it's hard to stay away from sweets, remember: it's only a few times a week that you have to say no, thank you.

Another plus is that giving up sugar several times a week will finally help you kill the sugar demon and get rid of this highly addictive substance.

Soft drinks (regular or diet), fruit juices, or sports drinks: Americans typically consume 140 to 180 calories per day through sugary drinks, such as carbonated drinks and sports drinks. Also avoid drinking the diet versions.

Alcohol: A 2012 study showed that, on average, Americans consume 300 calories per day from alcoholic beverages. This might seem less, but consider how much you can add in a week. In addition, many people consume a lot more each day.

A 5-ounce glass of red wine contains 125 calories. A regular 350ml beer has over 150 calories, and a double vodka and diet cola have 258 calories. Therefore, consuming just one of these drinks can dramatically lower calorie limits on fasting days.

Junk food including crisps, candies, pretzels, buttery popcorn, fruit snacks, etc.: One of the many pros of fasting is the cleansing ability it has on the body. Eating junk food, which is notoriously packed with nutritionally poor ingredients, on fasting days will only flush out the toxins you're trying to eliminate. Instead, opt for whole, natural foods, preferably unpackaged during fasting days.

A note on carbohydrates and sugar

There are no specific rules for how many grams of carbohydrate you can eat on the 5: 2 Fast Diet, but your fasting days should be low enough. It just means that you should get more carbs from vegetables than fruits and more fruits than grains. Sweets and desserts are allowed on days without fasting, but should be treats once a day or every other day.

One of the goals (and benefits) of intermittent fasting is to regulate insulin levels and insulin sensitivity. If you are eating too much simple carbohydrates, such as sugar, breads, and cereals on days without fasting, you are more likely to have spikes in blood sugar, which creates excess insulin in the bloodstream. Going from a high-carb day to a low-carb day (like fasting days) can make you more likely to develop insulin resistance. Insulin resistance, or metabolic syndrome, can cause excess belly fat, heart disease, and type 2 diabetes.

A note on drinks and hydration

Maintaining adequate hydration is very important for good health. This is especially important on the 5: 2 Fast Diet, as staying hydrated will help you feel less hungry, especially on fasting days.

You should drink a minimum of 64 fluid ounces of water per day! Some people find it easier if they freeze several bottles of water to carry around throughout the day. You can also pack multiple bottles in a cooler bag to take with you to work.

On fasting days, drinks are limited to:
- Unsweetened black coffee
- Water
- Unsweetened iced tea
- Unsweetened hot tea (without milk)

You will find that the 5: 2 Fast Diet is easy to adapt after just a few weeks, maybe even less. It is best to follow the menu plans we offer for fasting days for at least the first month, as calories have already been calculated and menus have been created to ensure a good balance of healthy carbohydrates, protein, nutrients and fats.

Once your body gets used to this healthier way of eating and you have a good idea of the right serving size and the types of foods you should be eating, feel free to create your own meal plans and use external recipes for your fasting days.

WHEN YOU SHOULD OR SHOULD NOT FAST ON THE 5:2 DIET

Before starting the 5: 2 diet or any other fast, talk to your doctor or health care professional about fasting, its benefits and harms, and your condition.

What times and days to fast?

The 5:2 diet suggests two days of modified fasting and five days without counting calories. When deciding which days of the week to fast, keep in mind that you may need to be flexible. What worked well for you last week may not work this week, due to social engagements or other obligations.

The key is to choose two non-consecutive days to fast. So, for instance, if you fasted on Monday, do not fast again until Wednesday or at the end of the week, allow an entire day between fasting periods .

If you decide to fast on Mondays and Thursdays of the week, now all you have to do is agree on the length of the fast. You will ideally fast for 16 hours at a time, which was considered the ideal fasting point - you get all the benefits of a longer fast without the difficulties of doing a longer fast (compared to a 24-hour fast)

But it can be difficult on the 5: 2 diet because you exceed your calorie limits between breakfast and dinner.

However, on fasting days you may find it easier to get all the calories from a meal. It really depends on you. The secret is to play with the fasting method you choose, but remember to follow a specific method for three months before trying a different one.

Three months is a great time to give your body a chance to respond to your chosen fasting method and see its results.

WHO MUST NOT TRY THE 5:2 DIET?

Some people should not fast on the 5:2 diet, including the following:

Pregnant Women: More research needs to be done to determine if fasting is harmless for pregnant women and, until experts prove that fasting is healthy during this time in their lives, do not fast.

Children: As children are still developing physically and mentally, they do not need nutritional stress.

Although occasional fasting helps reduce IGF-1 levels in adults (which helps promote general health and longevity), during the formative years of childhood, humans naturally have higher levels of IGF-1 to help them grow and develop properly. Never encourage people under 18 to fast.

People with health concerns: If you have underlying medical conditions, such as HIV/AIDS, cancer, diabetes, or an eating disorder, fasting is probably not a good choice.

If you are a fairly healthy adult looking to lose body fat, feel revitalized, and live a healthier lifestyle, the 5: 2 diet may be a viable option for you.

EXERCISE ON THE 5:2 FAST DIET

Exercise is essential for overall health and healthy weight loss. You can lose 3.5 pounds without exercise, but you still might not appreciate the results.

We've all seen thin men and women who looked soft, pale, and flabby. The goal of losing weight should be to look healthy and fit, and to feel strong and energized. This not only requires good nutrition, but also regular physical activity.

A comprehensive exercise program should include cardio and some form of weight training. Cardio helps burn calories, improves cardiovascular health, and may also help with hypertension and type 2 diabetes. Strength training maximizes lean muscle mass (which helps you burn more calories throughout the day), improves bone health and has been proved to improve longevity.

You should aim to do at least thirty minutes of cardiovascular activity three times a week and at least twenty minutes of strength training three times a week. These are the weak spots and you can definitely do more, but if your schedule is tight you can have a great workout in under thirty minutes.

Interval training for quick results in less time

Interval training is a way to get quick results in a very short period of time. Interval training is simply an alternation of periods of physical work. You can do this to combine strength training with cardio or use it just for cardio. For example:

- Do three to four sets of bench press, followed by two minutes of skipping rope, followed by three sets of barbell curls, and so on.
- Walk on level ground for five minutes, then climb two flights of stairs. Then walk on level ground for another five minutes, and so on.
- Alternate five rounds using the frog with five rounds using the back and so on.

High intensity interval training

HIIT (High Intensity Interval Training) is a variation of interval training that is much more effective, but also much more intense. It's cardio workout that can deliver incredible results in just a few minutes a day, but it's not for everyone.

With high-intensity interval training, you alternate short periods of very hard work with longer periods of more moderate work.

High intensity intervals are typically ten to thirty seconds long and moderate periods two to four minutes. Almost any cardiovascular activity can be adapted for high intensity interval training. You can run at a moderate pace for two minutes, run for thirty seconds, and then run again.

Repeat this pattern for about twenty minutes in total, starting and ending with a moderate period. You can also adapt HIIT for biking, climbing stairs, and many other cardiovascular activities where it's easy to change your pace.

HIIT has been shown to have a major impact on metabolism. You can expect to burn more calories (even at rest) for about 48 hours after a HIIT workout. Additionally, HIIT workouts typically burn as many calories in twenty minutes as sixty minutes of the same activity in the steady state version.

Whether you decide to do interval training or not, make sure you do at least three strength training exercises and three cardiovascular exercises per week. You may do it on the same day or every other day, but as you will read soon, strenuous exercise is not recommended on fasting days. Plan your workouts so that you can walk moderately or stretch on a brisk day. Cardio doesn't have to be difficult to be right for you.

Some good options for aerobic exercise are walking, swimming, cycling, dancing, and rowing. Strength training can be performed in our house or at the gym, with weight machines or dumbbells. You can also achieve a complete and effective workout by using bodyweight resistance movements like push-ups, push-ups, lunges, etc.

You may want to follow the first week or two of the 5: 2 Fast Diet before committing to a regular exercise program. It will be useful to understand more about how your body adapts to diet, how you feel on fasting days, and what times of day are best for you to train. Most people report better energy and strength levels when following an intermittent fasting diet, but they all adjust to the diet at their own pace. Until then, a thirty-minute walk or stretching exercises will still be good for your body.

Exercise on fasting days

While you've probably read or heard claims that you can continue to exercise even on fasting days, we don't recommend it, at least not in the first few weeks of the 5: 2 Fast Diet.

Our bodies are extremely adaptable mechanisms, but each body adapts to its own rhythm. While a person's metabolism may adjust more easily to stored energy intake (in the form of stored fat), others may take longer. This is due to differences in eating and exercise habits before starting the diet, as well as hormonal fluctuations.

On fasting days, you eat enough to work and even work well, but you may not have the energy stored in days without fasting or the fat stored to support intense training. The most positive outcome would be simply not having the energy or strength to perform training at a valid level. Even if you manage to get your workout done, you may feel much hungrier than you should afterwards.

The most serious effects of heavy training on fasting days can range from dizziness or feeling weak to muscle cramps or even injury.

On fasting days, we recommend that you exercise, but only at an easy or moderate level. This could mean swimming at a moderate pace, going for a thirty-minute walk, or doing yoga or stretching exercises.

Any physical activity is great for your body and will help you lose weight.

Continue your intense workouts for days without fasting and give your body a short break while fasting.

OTHER HEALTH BENEFITS OF THE 5:2 DIET

Even though many people undertake intermittent fasting and 5:2 fast diet to lose weight or to help you maintain your weight, there are many other health benefits. Since the goal of weight loss should not only be to look better, but also to improve overall health, these benefits should be considered as important as losing fat or wearing smaller clothes.

Research into the intermittent fasting effects is ongoing, but several studies indicate that intermittent fasting can have a significant impact on longevity, cognitive function, heart disease, and blood sugar— related issues such as metabolic syndrome and insulin sensitivity.

Insulin and Blood Sugar Benefits of Intermittent Fasting

In a 2005 study in Denmark, eight healthy men were placed on an alternating fasting regimen for fifteen days. At the end of the fortnight, the men showed a marked improvement in their sensitivity to insulin. The researchers explained that this improvement was linked to the "thrifty gene" theory which means that in Paleolithic times, humans often went days without eating, so our genes adapted to this feast or famine lifestyle.

In particular, certain hormones, like cortisol, stimulate the accumulation of fat to make us survive in times of lack of food.

The researchers noted that the abundance of food today keeps us from going through periods of fasting and this has contributed to the increase in metabolic syndrome or the combination of insulin resistance and obesity. They reported: "This experiment is the first in humans to show that intermittent fasting increases insulin-mediated glucose uptake rates and the results are consistent with the concept of a preservation gene."

This research is one of many that suggest that the fasting process is necessary to help regulate insulin sensitivity and the body's ability to use glucose for fuel instead of storing it as fat.

A 2011 study found that intermittent fasting had a positive impact on cholesterol and human growth hormone (HGH) levels.

The study found that intermittent fasting increased individuals' total cholesterol. LDL (low-density lipoprotein) or "bad" cholesterol has been increased by 14% and HDL (high-density lipoprotein) or "good" cholesterol has been increased by 6%. It might seem like a bad thing at first, but higher total cholesterol actually helps the body use fat for energy, which in turn reduces total body fat. The study clarified, "Fasting causes hunger or stress. In response, the body produces more cholesterol, that allows it to use fat for fuel instead of glucose. This minimizes the number of fat cells in the body, which is important because the less fat cells in a body, the less likely it is to suffer from insulin resistance or diabetes."

These researches are just the tip of the iceberg to show that intermittent fasting plans, like the 5: 2 Fast Diet, may have long-term benefits for insulin and blood sugar.

Intermittent fasting and heart disease

Reducing fat and regulating blood sugar and insulin levels are important steps in improving heart health. But some studies show that intermittent fasting can improve heart health and reduce the risk of coronary heart disease in other ways. In 2012, a study published in the American Journal of Cardiology found that periodic fasting can reduce the risk of type 2 diabetes and coronary heart disease. These results are promising for those looking to reduce the risk of heart disease through intermittent fasting.

Intermittent fasting and brain health

Intermittent fasting maximizes the production of the brain-derived neurotrophic factor (BDNF), a protein that stimulates the brain stem cells to become new neurons. It also protects brain cells from degenerative neurological diseases, such as Alzheimer's disease and Parkinson's disease. Intermittent fasting can increase the production of BDNF from 50 percent to 400 percent.

Everyone wants to be attractive, to feel fit and to be more confident in their skin. All of this can be accomplished with the help of the 5: 2 Fast Diet. However, the possible long term and very important health benefits can be considered as the main draw of the diet.

CHAPTER SEVEN: 5:2 FASTING DAY RECIPES

All of these fasting-day were created to make two servings. If you are the only one who follow the 5: 2 Fast Diet, simply split the recipe in half or reserve the second serving for another meal.

PARMESAN EGG TOAST WITH TOMATOES

150 calories per serving

This breakfast is quick to prepare and delicious to eat. You can substitute grape tomatoes if you have them on hand. They give your meal a healthy dose of vitamin C.

Ingredients

- ½ teaspoon chopped garlic (about 1 clove)
- 1 teaspoon olive oil
- 6 cherry tomatoes, quartered
- ¼ teaspoon freshly ground black pepper
- ½ teaspoon salt
- 2 large eggs
- 1 tablespoon shredded Parmesan cheese
- 2 Slices reduced-calorie whole wheat toast

Preparations

1. In a small skillet, preheat the oil over medium heat. Add the tomatoes and garlic into the pan and sauté for 2 minutes, stirring constantly. Season with salt and pepper and transfer to a plate to heat.
2. In the same pan, brown the eggs for 2 minutes. Flip and cook to desired point (30 seconds for very easy, 1 minute for medium, 2 minutes for very good).
3. Place one egg on the slices of toast, top with half the tomatoes and sprinkle with half the Parmesan.

GREEK BREAKFAST WRAPS

250 calories per serving

This recipe is as satisfying as the fast food breakfast sandwich, but this wrap has much less fat and fewer calories. It is a great morning coffee to make ahead of time and warm up in the morning or when you get to work.

Ingredients

- ½ cup fresh baby spinach leaves
- 1 teaspoon olive oil
- 1 tablespoon fresh basil
- ½ teaspoon salt
- 4 egg whites, beaten
- ¼ teaspoon freshly ground black pepper
- 2 (8-inch) whole wheat tortillas
- ¼ cup crumbed low-fat feta cheese

Preparation

1. In a small skillet, preheat the oil over medium heat. Add the basil and spinach to the pan and sauté for about 2 minutes or until the spinach wilts.
2. Add the egg whites to the pan, season with salt and pepper and sauté, stirring constantly, for another two minutes or until the egg whites are firm.
3. Remove from heat and sprinkle with feta cheese.
4. Microwave tortillas for 20 to 30 seconds, or until tender and warm. Divide the eggs between the tortillas and wrap them in a burrito style.

CURRIED CHICKEN BREAST WRAPS

250 calories per serving

These quick and filling wraps deliver lots of flavor with very few calories. Make the filling ahead of time to have on hand for work lunches and busy days.

Ingredients

- 2 tablespoons plain low-fat yogurt

- 6 ounces cooked chicken breast, cubed
- 1 teaspoon Dijon mustard
- 1 small Gala or Granny Smith apple, cored and chopped
- ½ teaspoon mild curry powder
- 1 cup spring lettuce mix or baby lettuce
- 2 (8-inch) whole wheat tortillas

Preparations

1. In a small bowl, combine the yogurt, chicken, Dijon mustard and curry powder; mix well to combine. Add the apple and mix well.
2. Divide the lettuce between the tortillas and add the chicken mixture to each half. Wrap in a burrito shape and serve.

PROTEIN POWER SWEET POTATOES

200 calories per serving

This recipe is extremely simple and quick, yet it has almost ten grams of protein per serving, making it a perfect fasting meal to keep you satisfied and help keep you energized and focused.

Ingredients

- ½ teaspoon salt

- 2 medium sweet potatoes
- ¼ teaspoon freshly ground black pepper
- 1/3 Cup dried cranberries
- 6 ounces plain Greek yogurt

Preparations

1. Preheat the oven to 400°F and pierce the sweet potatoes a few times with a fork. Put it on a baking sheet then bake for 40 to 45 minutes or until they bite easily with a fork.
2. Cut the potatoes in half and pour the pulp into a medium bowl, keeping the skins intact. Add salt, pepper, yogurt and cranberries to the bowl and mix well with a fork.
3. Pour the mixture into the potato skin and serve hot.

BAKED SALMON FILLETS WITH TOMATO AND MUSHROOMS

200 calories per serving

Salmon is a good source of healthy fats, especially omega-3 fatty acids. When cooked with a mixture of spicy tomatoes and sweet mushrooms, it is as delicious as it is healthy.

Ingredients

- 2 teaspoons olive oil, divided
- 2 (4-ounce) skin-on salmon fillets

- ½ teaspoon salt
- ½ teaspoon chopped fresh dill
- ¼ teaspoon freshly ground black pepper
- ½ cup diced fresh tomato
- ½ cup sliced fresh mushrooms

Preparations

1. Preheat the oven to 375°F and line a baking sheet with foil.
2. Making use of a pastry brush or your fingers, coat both sides of the fillets with ½ teaspoon of olive oil each. Place the salmon skin face down in the pan. Sprinkle evenly with salt and pepper.
3. In a bowl, combine the remaining teaspoon of olive oil, dill, tomato and mushrooms; mix well to combine. Pour the mixture over the fillets.
4. Fold the foil sides and ends to seal the fish, place the pan on the middle oven rack and bake it for about 20 minutes or until the salmon comes off easily.

AVOCADO AND FENNEL SALAD WITH BALSAMIC VINAIGRETTE

150 calories per serving

This salad is a wonderful blend of spicy citrus, silky avocado and herbs - sweet with an anise flavor. Played with a quick and easy balsamic vinaigrette, it's perfect for lunch or light dinner for warm days.

Ingredients

- 1 tablespoon balsamic vinegar
- 1 tablespoon light olive oil
- ¼ teaspoon salt
- ½ avocado, diced
- ½ cup fennel, sliced
- ½ cup mandarin oranges, drained
- ¼ teaspoon freshly ground black pepper
- 1 cup chopped romaine lettuce

Preparation

1. Combine balsamic vinegar, olive oil, pepper and salt in a small bowl and beat until smooth and slightly thickened. Here is your balsamic vinaigrette.
2. Add the fennel, avocado, orange and lettuce; stir until vegetables are well coated with seasoning. Divide between two salad plates and serve cold.

HEARTY SHRIMP AND KALE SOUP

250 calories per serving

This tasty soup packs abundance of antioxidants from the kale and carrots, in addition to a healthy amount of protein comes from the beans and shrimp. It is simple, delicious, and satisfying.

Ingredients

- 2 Cloves garlic
- 1 teaspoon olive oil
- ¼ cup chopped onion
- 1 cup thinly sliced fresh carrots
- 2 Cups chopped fresh kale
- ½ teaspoon salt
- 8 medium (36–40 count) raw shrimp, peeled and halved
- 1½ cups vegetable stock
- 1 cup canned great northern beans, drained
- ¼ teaspoon freshly ground black pepper
- ¼ cup chopped fresh parsley

Preparations

1. Heat the oil over little heat in a small saucepan. Add the garlic, onion, cabbage and carrots and sauté for 5 minutes, stirring constantly.
2. Season the veggies with pepper and salt and add the vegetable broth. Cook uncovered for 30 minutes or until carrots are tender.
3. Increase the heat and let the soup boil. Add the shrimp and cook 2 minutes or until the shrimp are pink and slightly firm. Reduce the heat.
4. Use a fork to knead about a quarter of the beans. Mix all the beans in the soup and add the parsley. Cook 2 minutes or until completely hot.
5. Put the ladle into the bowls and serve hot.

PENNE PASTA WITH VEGETABLES

200 calories per serving

Even on fasting days, you can enjoy a light meal of pasta. This one is chock-full of iron and vitamin C from the tomatoes and spinach and delivers lots of flavor and satisfaction.

Ingredients

- ¾ cup uncooked penne pasta
- 1 teaspoon salt, divided
- 1 tablespoon olive oil
- 1 teaspoon chopped fresh oregano
- 1 tablespoon chopped garlic
- 1 cup sliced fresh mushrooms
- 1 cup fresh spinach leaves
- 10 cherry tomatoes, halved
- ½ teaspoon freshly ground black pepper
- 1 tablespoon shredded Parmesan cheese

Preparations

1. In a medium saucepan, bring one liter of water to a boil. Add ½ teaspoon of salt and penne and cook according to package directions or al dente (about 9 minutes). Drain, but do not rinse the penne, reserving about ¼ cup of water for the pasta.

2. Meanwhile, in a large skillet, heat the oil over medium-high heat. Add the garlic, oregano and mushrooms and sauté for 4 to 5 minutes or until the mushrooms are golden brown.
3. Add the season, tomatoes and spinach with the remaining ½ teaspoon of salt and pepper and sauté for three to four mins or until the spinach wilts.
4. Add the drained pasta to the pot, as well as 2-3 tablespoons of water for the pasta. Cook, stirring continuously, two to three mins or until the dough is shiny and the water is cooked through.
5. Divide the dough into two shallow bowls and sprinkle with Parmesan cheese. Serve hot or at room temperature.

PORK LOIN CHOPS WITH MANGO SALSA

250 calories per serving

This recipe is full of flavor and satisfying enough to make you forget you are fasting. The sauce is even better. Prepare a day ahead and marinate in the refrigerator overnight with pork chops.

Ingredients

- ½ cup lime juice
- 2 pork loin chops, ¾ inch thick
- Juice of 1 large orange
- ½ cup diced green bell pepper
- 1 large ripe mango, peeled and diced

- ½ cup diced red bell pepper
- 1 tablespoon chopped fresh cilantro
- 1 small jalapeño pepper, seeded and diced
- ½ cup diced red onion
- ½ teaspoon salt
- 1 tbn chopped fresh parsley
- ¼ tbn freshly ground black pepper

Preparations

1. Place the pork chops in the freezer and add the lemon and orange juice. Seal, shake to mix well and refrigerate overnight.
2. In a bowl, combine the mango, red onion, peppers, jalapeño, cilantro and parsley. Stir to mix well. Cover and refrigerate overnight.
3. Preheat broiler and line a baking sheet of aluminum foil.
4. Season the pork chops on each sides with pepper and salt. Put in the pot and cook 4-5 minutes on one side, turn and cook another 4-5 minutes. Place the pork chops on a different plate, drizzle with sauce and serve.

SPINACH AND SWISS CHEESE OMELETTE

150 calories per serving

It is not necessary to reserve omelette for breakfast or brunch. An omelette can be a great dining option on busy nights and is also a good appetizer for lunch on weekends.

Ingredients

- 6 large egg whites, beaten
- 1 teaspoon olive oil
- 1 cup fresh baby spinach leaves
- ¼ teaspoon freshly ground black pepper
- ½ teaspoon salt
- 2 (1-ounce) slices reduced-fat Swiss cheese

Preparations

1. Preheat the oil over high heat in a small skillet. Add the spinach, salt and pepper and brown for 3 minutes, stirring constantly.
2. Use a spatula to spread the spinach evenly over the bottom of the pan and pour the egg whites on top, tilting the pan to completely cover the spinach.
3. Cook for 3-4 minutes, occasionally pulling the edges of the eggs towards the center while tilting the saucepan to allow the raw egg to spread over the edges of the pan.
4. When the center of the eggs is almost (but not completely) dry, use a spatula to turn the eggs. Place the Swiss cheese slices in one half of the omelet and turn the other half to form a half moon. Cook until cheese is melted and heated through.
5. To serve, cut the omelet in half and serve hot.

LEMON-SESAME CHICKEN AND ASPARAGUS

200 calories per serving

Chicken and asparagus go together well, and this recipe combines them with a hint of lemon and the added crunch of sesame seeds.

Ingredients

- ½ cup plus 1 tablespoon lemon juice, divided
- 8 ounces skinless chicken breast tenders (or quartered chicken breast)
- 1 teaspoon chopped fresh rosemary
- ½ teaspoon olive oil
- 6 medium spears fresh asparagus, cut into 2-inch pieces
- 1 teaspoon salt, divided
- 2 tablespoons sesame seeds
- ¼ teaspoon freshly ground black pepper

Preparations

1. Beat the chicken slices with a hammer or the palm of your hand until they are evenly ½ inch thick. Place in the freezer with ½ cup of lemon juice and marinate for 2 hours or overnight.
2. Preheat grill and line a baking sheet of aluminum foil.

3. Season the chicken on both sides with ½ teaspoon of salt and pepper and place in the pan. Sprinkle with rosemary.
4. In a small bowl, season the asparagus with the oil, the remaining tablespoon of lemon juice and the remaining ½ teaspoon of salt. Arrange the asparagus around the chicken in the pan.
5. Grill the chicken for 4 to 5 minutes, turn it over and add the asparagus and cook for another 4 to 5 minutes.
6. Divide the chicken and asparagus between two plates and sprinkle with the sesame seeds.

GRILLED CHICKEN SALAD WITH POPPY SEED SAUCE

200 calories per serving

Salads are easy to prepare, and when prepared with lots of fresh, high-fiber vegetables, they provide lots of nourishment with very few calories. This salad not only tastes nice, but also fills us up really well.

Ingredients

- 1 tablespoon apple cider vinegar
- 2 tablespoons light olive oil
- 1 teaspoon Dijon mustard
- ½ cup chopped cooked chicken breast
- 1 tablespoon poppy seeds
- 1 cup chopped romaine lettuce

- 1 medium red bell pepper, chopped
- 1 medium unpeeled cucumber, sliced
- 1 small red onion, chopped

Preparations

1. In a bowl, combine Dijon mustard, olive oil, apple cider vinegar and poppy seeds for about 1 minute or until combined and well blended.
2. Add the chicken, lettuce, cucumber, peppers and onions and mix well until smooth.
3. Divide between two salad plates and serve immediately.

TOASTED PEPPER JACK SANDWICHES

150 calories per serving

Toast instead of grilling your cheese sandwich adds tons of satisfying crunch while omitting unnecessary fat. These toasted cheese sandwiches have a very spicy flavor in every bite.

Ingredients

- 4 slices reduced-calorie whole wheat bread
- 2 Slices reduced-calorie pepper jack cheese
- ½ cup fresh arugula leaves
- 4 thin slices fresh tomato

Preparations

1. Preheat the oven to 350 degrees F.
2. Place one slice of cheese on the 2 slices of bread; decorate each with 2 slices of tomato and half of the arugula. Cover with the rest of the slices of bread and place the buns on a baking sheet in the center of the oven.
3. Broil for 4 minutes, then flip and toast for an additional 2-3 minutes, or until bread is golden and cheese is melted. Cut each loaf in half to serve.

BROILED HALIBUT WITH GARLIC SPINACH

200 calories per serving

Halibut is a deliciously moist fish loaded with healthy omega-3 fatty acids. If you substitute frozen halibut, be sure to thaw it completely and pat it very dry before cooking.

Ingredients

- ½ lemon (about 1 teaspoon juice)
- 2 (4-ounce) halibut fillets, 1 inch thick
- 1 teaspoon salt, divided
- ½ teaspoon cayenne pepper
- ¼ teaspoon freshly ground black pepper
- 1 teaspoon olive oil

- ½ cup chopped red onion
- 2 Cloves garlic
- 2 Cups fresh baby spinach leaves

Preparation

1. Preheat the grill and place an oven rack 4 to 5 inches below the heat source. Line a baking sheet with foil.
2. Squeeze half the lemon over the fish fillets and season each side with ½ teaspoon of salt, pepper and cayenne pepper. Place the fish in the pan and grill for 7-8 minutes. Flip the fish and grill for another 6 to 7 minutes or until chipped.
3. Meanwhile, heat the oil in a skillet. Add the garlic and onion then sauté for 2 minutes. Add the spinach and the remaining ½ teaspoon of salt and sauté for another 2 minutes. Remove from heat then cover to keep warm.
4. To serve, divide the spinach into two plates and decorate each serving with a fish fillet. Serve hot.

QUICK MISO SOUP WITH SHRIMP AND BOK CHOY

150 calories per serving

If you like Asian flavors, you are going to love this quick, simple soup. It become ready in just a few minutes which makes it a great recipe for the busiest nights. It reheats well, so it's also a good option for a weekday lunch.

Ingredients

- 8 large (34–40 count) raw shrimp, peeled and halved
- 2 Cups water
- 1 cup chopped bok choy
- 1 cup cubed firm tofu
- ¼ cup white miso paste
- 2 green onions, chopped

Preparations

1. In a saucepan, boil the water over high heat. Add the shrimp and allow to boil for one minute.
2. Reduce the heat and add the bok choy. Cook for 2 minutes, then add the miso and tofu. Cook for another minute.
3. To serve, divide into two bowls and sprinkle with chives.

QUINOA WITH SWEET POTATOES AND CURRIED BLACK BEANS

250 calories per serving

The beans, quinoa and sweet potato combine to provide a filling and healthy portion of meatless protein which is very satisfying.

You can prepare quinoa in the microwave if you prefer; just follow the directions on the package to get a cup.

Ingredients

- 1 cup water
- ½ cup quinoa
- ½ cup diced and peeled sweet potato (about 1 small)
- ½ teaspoon dried rosemary
- ½ teaspoon olive oil
- 1 cup canned black beans, drained
- 2 tablespoons chopped fresh parsley
- 1 teaspoon mild curry powder

Preparations

1. Wash the quinoa under cold running water through a fine mesh sieve. Drain well on absorbent paper then dry.
2. In a small saucepan, toast the quinoa for 2 minutes over medium heat, stirring constantly. Add the water, heat and let it boil. Cover, reduce heat and cook 15 minutes or until it as quinoa is plump and the germ as small spirals in each grain. Remove from heat then cover to keep warm.
3. In a small bowl, season the sweet potatoes with olive oil and rosemary. Transfer to a medium skillet over medium-high heat. Sauté, stirring constantly, for 6 to 7 minutes or until well caramelized. Add the black beans and curry powder, reduce the heat to medium and cook, stirring constantly, until the beans are heated through.

4. To serve, place ½ cup of cooked quinoa on each plate and top with half the bean mixture. Garnish with parsley.

CHAPTER EIGHT: HEALTHY RECIPES FOR NON-FASTING DAYS

The recipes for the non-fasting days are low in calories, but suitable for guests or the whole family, so we created most of them to make four servings. If you want, you may slice the ingredients in half or freeze additional portions for easy reheating the next day.

BREAKFAST

SALMON AND TOMATO EGG SANDWICHES

This sandwich breakfast is much healthier and more important than all that you can pick up at the drive-through; It is also very tasty, but it only takes a few minutes to prepare.

Ingredients

- 1 teaspoon olive oil
- 4 light multigrain English muffins
- 6 ounces canned pink salmon
- 8 large eggs, beaten
- 1 cup diced tomatoes
- ½ teaspoon salt
- 1 cup fresh arugula
- ¼ teaspoon freshly ground black pepper

Preparations

1. Toast English muffins while preparing eggs.
2. In a skillet, heat the oil. Add the salmon and tomatoes to the pan and sauté, stirring constantly, for 4 minutes.
3. Pour over eggs, season with salt and pepper and stir, stirring constantly, for about 2 minutes or until eggs solidify.
4. Place English muffin halves on 4 plates and cover each bottom half with a quarter of the egg mixture. Complete with the rocket and the other half of the muffin.

NUTTY PEACH PARFAITS

These parfaits may look good, but are also healthier than they look. The walnuts add omega-3 fats and fiber as well as crunch, and the Greek yogurt has as much as fourteen grams of protein per cup.

Ingredients

- 4 (6-ounce) containers vanilla Greek yogurt
- 4 medium peaches, sliced
- ½ cup unsalted walnuts, chopped

Preparation

1. Divide the ingredients between four parfaits or desserts. Start with a layer of peaches; then add a spoonful of yogurt and a pinch of walnuts.

COCOA-BANANA BREAKFAST SMOOTHIE

This smoothie only takes seconds to prepare, but is packed with healthy nutrients. Greek yogurt provides a dose of protein, and bananas are a great source of potassium.

Ingredients

- 2 medium bananas, cut into chunks
- 24 ounces vanilla Greek yogurt
- 1 teaspoon honey
- ½ cup low-fat milk
- 2 tablespoons unsweetened cocoa powder
- ½ cup ice cubes

Preparation

1. Place the yogurt and bananas in a blender and blend until smooth. Add honey, cocoa and milk and beat again until combined.
2. Add ice and beat again, pulsing as needed, until smooth and thick.

SCRAMBLED EGG SOFT TACOS

Finding fast food alternatives for your morning meal can be difficult, but this recipe is great to try. It's packed with Southwestern flavors, but low in fat and calories.

Ingredients

- 1 teaspoon olive oil
- 8 (6-inch) whole wheat tortillas
- 2 green onions, chopped
- 12 large eggs, beaten
- ½ teaspoon cayenne pepper
- 1 cup mild chunky salsa
- 1 cup low-fat shredded cheddar cheese

Preparations

1. Put the tortillas on a plate, then cover with a damp paper towel and microwave for about one mins, or until warm and supple. Cover with a second dish or a pan lid to keep them warm.
2. In a big, heavy-bottomed pan, heat the oil over medium heat. Add the chives and sauté for 1 minute. Add the cayenne pepper to the eggs and place them in the pan. Stir, stirring constantly, until eggs are cooked through, about 5 minutes.

3. Divide the egg mixture evenly between the tortillas, decorate the tortillas with 2 tablespoons of salsa and cheddar cheese and fold the tacos in half.

CRANBERRY-WALNUT WHOLE WHEAT PANCAKES

These pancakes are a delightful way to start the day. Blueberries are sour, but sweet, and the nuts add crunch and texture to this comfort classic.

Ingredients

- ¾ cup whole wheat flour
- ½ cup fresh cranberries
- 2 tablespoons sugar
- ¼ teaspoon salt
- 1 tablespoon baking powder
- ½ teaspoon ground nutmeg
- 1¼ cup low-fat milk
- ½ teaspoon pure vanilla extract
- 1 large egg, beaten
- 1 tablespoon coconut oil, divided
- ½ cup chopped walnuts

Preparations

1. In a bowl, toss the cranberries with a handful of wholemeal flour, turning them well to coat.
2. In a bowl, combine the remaining flour, sugar, baking powder, salt and nutmeg, stirring to combine well.
3. Add the egg, vanilla, milk and mix well, but without stirring too much. The dough should remain a little uneven. Gently mix the nuts and cranberries (with the flour) and set the dough aside for 10 minutes.
4. In a large, heavy-bottomed pan, heat about ½ teaspoon of coconut oil over medium heat. Mix enough batter in the pan to make a 6 inch pancake. Cook until the edges are bubbling, then flip the pancake and cook for another minute. Transfer to a plate then cover it to keep warm while making the rest of the pancakes. Add extra coconut oil to the pan as needed.
5. To serve, place 2 pancakes on each plate and decorate with hot maple syrup, honey or molasses.

HERB AND SWISS FRITTATA

This frittata looks like something you'd see in a restaurant, but it only takes a few minutes to get ready. You'll love the layered flavors, thanks to the sweet Swiss cheese and fresh herbs.

Ingredients

- 8 large eggs, beaten
- 2 teaspoons olive oil
- ½ teaspoon salt

- 2 teaspoons chopped fresh parsley
- ½ teaspoon freshly ground black pepper
- 2 teaspoons chopped fresh marjoram
- ½ cup shredded low-fat Swiss cheese
- 1 teaspoon chopped fresh basil

Preparation

1. Preheat the oven to 375 degrees F.
2. Heat oil on a large baking sheet over high heat. Pour the eggs, distributing them evenly on the baking sheet. Season with salt and pepper.
3. Take down the pan from the heat and sprinkle the parsley, marjoram and basil evenly over the eggs. Cover with Swiss cheese.
4. Place the pan in the oven center and bake for 18 to 25 minutes or until a toothpick you inserted in the center is clean.
5. To serve, cut into four slices and serve hot.

SCRAMBLED EGGS WITH MUSHROOMS AND ONIONS

This egg dish cooks fast, but has a flavor that will require you to take it slowly and taste it. It's also a great sandwich filling. If you must grab your breakfast on the go, a whole pita pocket is a good choice.

Ingredients

- 1 cup sliced fresh mushrooms
- 1 teaspoon olive oil
- ¼ cup thinly sliced yellow onion
- ½ cup chopped fresh parsley
- 1 tablespoon chopped fresh tarragon
- ½ teaspoon salt
- 8 large eggs, beaten
- ½ teaspoon freshly ground black pepper

Preparations

1. In a heavy-bottomed pan, heat the oil. Add the mushrooms, onion, tarragon, parsley, salt and pepper and sauté for 4 minutes, stirring occasionally.
2. Pour in the eggs and stir, stirring constantly, until cooked through, about 2 minutes. To serve, divide into 4 plates.

VANILLA-ALMOND PROTEIN SHAKE

This breakfast shake contains lots of healthy proteins and fats to keep you going on even your toughest mornings. It's a great way to make breakfast - just pour it into a travel mug and drink it on the go.

Ingredients

- 4 scoops unflavored whey protein isolate powder
- 2 Cups cold water
- ¼ cup almond butter
- ½ teaspoon almond extract

- 2 tablespoons honey
- ½ teaspoon ground nutmeg
- 10 ice cubes

Preparations

1. In a blender, combine cold water, protein powder, almond butter, honey, almond extract, and nutmeg. Beat over high heat for about 30 seconds or until smooth.
2. Add ice cubes and beat again until thick and creamy. Drink immediately.

GRILLED FRUIT SALAD

Fruits don't always have to be raw; in fact, toasting or grilling fresh fruit enhances its natural sugars and enhances its flavor. Duplicate the recipe and use the leftovers as a side dish for chicken or seafood.

Ingredients

- 4 fresh peaches or nectarines, pitted and sliced into 8 pieces each
- 8 slices fresh or canned (unsweetened) pineapple
- 8 (½- inch-thick) slices fresh honeydew melon
- ½ teaspoon salt
- 1 teaspoon honey, warmed for 30 seconds in microwave

Preparations

1. Preheat the grill then line a baking sheet with foil.
2. Spread the fruit in one single layer on the baking sheet and brush with honey on both sides. Sprinkle salt on top and place the pan 3 cm under the grill.
3. Cook 3 minutes, turn each piece of fruit and cook for another 2 minutes, or until the fruit is somewhat browned around the edges.
4. Place 2 pineapple slices, 8 peach slices and 2 melon slices on each of the 4 plates and serve hot.

EASY GRANOLA BARS

This recipe is much greater for you than any other commercial cereal bars, which are often laden with less healthy grains and high-fructose corn syrup. These bars baked up in a snap and can be stored in an airtight container for up to a week, or if they last that long.

Ingredients

- 1 cup pecan pieces
- 1 teaspoon coconut oil
- 1 cup raw pumpkin seeds
- 1 cup dried cranberries
- 1 cup chopped walnuts
- 1 cup dried apricots, chopped
- ¼ cup coconut oil, melted

- 1 cup unsweetened coconut flakes
- ½ cup almond butter
- ¼ teaspoon pure vanilla extract
- 1 teaspoon ground cinnamon
- ½ cup raw honey
- ½ teaspoon salt

Preparations

1. Preheat the oven to 325 °F. Grease a 9 by 13-inch baking dish with 1 teaspoon of coconut oil and set aside.
2. In a large bowl, combine walnuts, pumpkin seeds, walnuts, cranberries, apricots, and coconut flakes and mix well.
3. In a pan, mix the melted coconut oil, almond butter, honey, vanilla, salt and cinnamon and heat until the honey is melted.
4. Transfer the nut mixture into the baking sheet, pressing down to distribute it evenly. Pour the honey mixture calmly over the top.
5. Bake until golden brown (40 to 45 mins). Allow the mixture to cool to room temperature before cutting it into equal bars. Store in an airtight vessel for up to 1 week.

HEARTY HOT CEREAL WITH BERRIES

Whole grains aren't only good for your heart; they are also perfect for your life. The content which is high in fiber makes them filling and provides a slow and sustained energy for your day. The addition of red fruits and nuts to this recipe makes it particularly satisfying.

Ingredients

- ½ teaspoon salt
- 4 cups water
- 2 tablespoons honey
- 2 Cups whole rolled oats
- ½ cup fresh blueberries
- ½ cup fresh raspberries
- 1 cup low-fat milk
- ½ cup chopped walnuts
- 2 teaspoons flaxseed

Preparations

1. In a saucepan, boil the water over high heat and add salt.
2. Add the oats, nuts and flax seeds, reduce the heat and cover. Cook for 20 minutes or until oats reach desired consistency.
3. Divide the oats among 4 deep bowls and cover each with 2 tablespoons of blueberries and raspberries. Add ¼ cup of milk to each bowl and serve.

PECAN-BANANA POPS

A healthy breakfast doesn't have to be hot; in fact, this one is frozen. Make a few of these pops ahead of time and keep them in the freezer. They are also a great after school gift. Kids love them!

Ingredients

- 2 tablespoons raw honey
- 4 large just-ripe bananas
- 4 Popsicle sticks
- ¾ cup chopped pecans
- ½ cup almond butter

Preparations

1. Peel and cut one end of each banana and insert a popsicle stick into the cut end.
2. In a bowl, mix the almond butter and honey and heat in the microwave for until the mixture is slightly diluted. Pour over a sheet of baking paper or aluminum foil and spread with a spatula.
3. On another piece of parchment paper or plastic wrap, spread the chopped nuts. Line a plate or sheet with a third piece of parchment paper or plastic wrap.
4. Wrap each banana first in the honey mixture until well coated, then in the nuts until completely coated, pressing gently so that the nuts stick together.
5. Place each ready-made banana on the baking sheet. When all the bananas are covered, place the dough in the freezer for at least 2 hours. For long-term storage, transfer the frozen bananas to a resealable plastic bag.

LUNCH

The recipes for the non-fasting days are low in calories, but suitable for guests or the whole family, so we created most of them to make four servings. If you want, you may divide the ingredients in half or freeze additional portions for easy reheating the next day.

TUNA AND BEAN SALAD POCKETS

This light yet hearty recipe is perfect for workday lunches. It packs well and tastes better because you have the option of sitting down, so make your salad the night before and put it in your pita pocket, then in your lunch box in the morning.

Ingredients

- 1 (6-ounce) can tuna filled in water, drained
- 4 whole wheat pita pockets
- ½ (15-ounce) can pinto beans, rinsed and drained
- 2 tablespoons light mayonnaise
- ¼ cup diced white onion
- 1 teaspoon spicy brown mustard
- ½ teaspoon freshly ground black pepper
- ½ teaspoon celery seed
- 1 cup chopped romaine lettuce

Preparations

1. If the rolls are not sliced, cut them so that there is a pocket-like opening, being careful not to cut the sides or the bottom.
2. In a small bowl, combine the tuna, borlotti beans, onion, mayonnaise, mustard, celery and pepper; mix well.
3. Divide the lettuce among the pita pockets and top each with a quarter of the tuna salad.

SHRIMP AND CRANBERRY SALAD

Dried cranberries add a tangy touch of flavor to this fresh shrimp salad. Using steamed shrimp from your seafood counter makes this a really quick lunch to make.

Ingredients

- ½ cup sliced red onion
- 1 dozen large (26–30 count) cooked shrimp, peeled and deveined
- ¼ cup lime juice
- ¼ teaspoon paprika
- ¼ teaspoon ground cumin
- 2 Cups chopped romaine lettuce
- ½ orange bell pepper, chopped
- ½ yellow bell pepper, chopped
- ¼ cup dried cranberries
- ¼ cup of your favorite homemade or store-bought balsamic vinaigrette

Preparations

1. In a small bowl, season the shrimp with the lemon juice, cumin and paprika and let stand 30 minutes in the refrigerator. Then drain.
2. In a large bowl, combine lettuce, onion, peppers and cranberries until smooth.
3. Add the marinated shrimp and balsamic vinaigrette and toss again. Divide among 4 salad plates and serve.

CHICKEN BREAST WITH ROASTED SUMMER VEGGIES

This recipe reheats really well, so make it on the weekend or at night and wrap it in individual containers to take out for lunch during the week. Experiment with other seasonal vegetables to vary the flavors.

Ingredients

- 1 tbn plus 1 teaspoon olive oil, divided
- 4 (4-to 5-ounce) skinless chicken breasts
- 1 teaspoon salt, divided
- ½ teaspoon ground turmeric
- ½ teaspoon freshly ground black pepper, divided
- 1 medium zucchini, thinly sliced
- 1 medium white onion, sliced ½ inch thick
- 2 yellow squash, thinly sliced
- 1 pint cherry tomatoes

- 1 teaspoon dried oregano
- 1 teaspoon dried parsley

Preparations

1. Preheat the oven to 400°F and line a baking pan with aluminum foil.
2. Rub each sides of the chicken breasts with 1 teaspoon of the olive oil and season them with ½ teaspoon of the salt, ¼ teaspoon of the pepper, and the turmeric. Place the chicken on the pan.
3. In a bowl, combine the squash, zucchini, onion, and tomatoes. Add the parsley and oregano and then drizzle with the remaining 1 tablespoon olive oil. Toss the vegetables well until they are evenly coated, and spread around the chicken breasts on the pan.
4. Bake in the oven center for 15 minutes, turn over the chicken and stir the vegetables, and then bake for 12 minutes more, or until the chicken juices run clear.
5. To serve, place 1 breast on each plate and top with one-quarter of the vegetables.

SEAFOOD-STUFFED AVOCADOES

This is a great light lunch, especially during the warmer months. You can prepare the filling up to three days ahead and just assemble the dish when you're ready to eat.

Ingredients

- 1 cup cooked cocktail shrimp
- 2 tablespoons light mayonnaise
- 8 ounces imitation flaked crabmeat, chopped
- 1 tablespoon plain yogurt
- 1 stalk celery, finely chopped
- ½ red bell pepper, chopped
- ½ red onion, chopped
- 2 SCallions, sliced
- ¼ teaspoon dry mustard
- 2 tablespoons chopped fresh parsley
- ½ teaspoon freshly ground black pepper
- 2 avocados
- 1 teaspoon lemon juice

Preparations

1. In a mixing bowl, combine the shrimp, crabmeat, celery, bell pepper, onion, and scallions; mix well.
2. In a bowl, combine the yogurt, mayonnaise, dry mustard, parsley, and black pepper, and stir with a fork until well combined.
3. Combine the mayonnaise mixture with the seafood filling until well blended.
4. Cut the avocados into half, remove the pits, and wipe the flesh with the lemon juice. Fill each avocado half with one-quarter of the seafood filling and serve.

EASY CHICKEN PASTA SOUP

Boil the pasta a day or two ahead of time and after draining, place it in a resealable bag in the fridge until it is ready to use. This bit of prep work Makes this soup a lunch that takes just ten minutes to make.

Ingredients

- 3 Cups chicken stock
- 1 cup frozen green beans
- 1 cup frozen sliced carrots
- 1 (6-ounce) can flaked chicken, drained
- 1 teaspoon chopped fresh tarragon
- 1 teaspoon fresh thyme leaves
- ½ teaspoon salt
- ¼ teaspoon freshly ground black pepper
- 1 cup cooked mini-shell pasta
- ½ cup shredded Parmesan cheese

Preparations

1. In a pan, boil the chicken stock over high heat. Add the green beans and carrots, and reduce the heat to medium. Cover and let simmer for 5 minutes.
2. Add the chicken, tarragon, thyme, salt, and pepper, and simmer for 4 minutes more. Put down the pan from the heat and stir in the cooked pasta.
3. To serve, divide between 4 bowls and top with the Parmesan.

CHOPPED BLT SALAD

This salad lets you enjoy all the flavors of the classic BLT sandwich without going overboard on fat and calories. Using turkey bacon and croutons (instead of bread) go a long way toward making this a healthier way to have a BLT.

Ingredients

- 4 slices turkey bacon
- 2 Cups chopped iceberg lettuce
- 2 medium tomatoes, diced
- ½ cup plain croutons
- 1 tablespoon mayonnaise
- 1 tablespoon light Italian dressing

Preparations

1. Prepare the turkey bacon in the microwave according to package directions. Allow it to drain on paper towels and cool for 5 minutes.
2. Meanwhile, combine the lettuce, tomatoes, and croutons in a large bowl.
3. In a small cup, stir together the mayonnaise and Italian dressing (it will be thick).
4. Crush the bacon and add to the salad. Pour the dressing over all and stir well until the salad is well coated. Divide between 2 plates and serve.

TOASTED HAM, SWISS, AND ARUGULA SANDWICHES

This toasted sandwich omits the fat of the typical grilled ham and cheese and adds a lot more crunch. Served with a light soup or a salad, this is a delicious and healthy lunchtime meal.

Ingredients

- 8 slices reduced-calorie whole wheat bread
- 2 teaspoons Dijon mustard
- 1 pound (about 16 slices) thinly sliced lean deli ham
- 8 slices reduced-fat Swiss cheese
- 1 cup fresh arugula

Preparations

1. Preheat the oven to 350 degrees F.
2. Separate four slices of the bread with the Dijon mustard, and top with about 4 slices of ham and 2 Slices of cheese.
3. Top each with ¼ cup arugula and place the remaining bread slices onto the sandwiches. Bake in the oven center for 5 minutes, turn over, and then bake until the cheese is melted and the bread is golden. Divide each sandwich in half and serve hot.

POWER-PACKED GREEN SMOOTHIE

Even if you don't have time for Much of a lunch, you'll still have time to get a heaping helping of minerals and vitamins in the form of this smoothie. The healthy fat from the avocado and the fiber from the vegetables Mean you'll feel satisfied, too.

Ingredients

- 1 medium cucumber, peeled and chopped
- 2 Cups fresh baby spinach
- ½ cup fresh parsley
- 1 cup carrot juice
- ½ teaspoon salt
- 2 dashes red pepper hot sauce
- ½ avocado, chopped

Preparations

1. Combine the cucumber, spinach, parsley, carrot juice, salt, and hot sauce in a blender and blend on high until smooth.
2. Add the avocado and blend on medium speed until smooth. Divide between 4 glasses and serve immediately.

QUICK AND LIGHT WHITE BEAN CHILI

This chili takes no time (and only one pan) to cook, and it tastes even better the next day. It also freezes well, so ensure to make a double batch to portion and store in the freezer for busy days.

Ingredients

- 1 teaspoon olive oil
- 1 pound freshly ground turkey breast
- 1 teaspoon chili powder
- 1 teaspoon salt
- ½ tsn freshly ground black pepper
- ½ teaspoon ground cumin
- 1 cup diced white onion
- 2 tablespoons chopped fresh cilantro
- 2 (15-ounce) cans great northern beans, undrained
- 2 Cups chicken stock

Preparations

1. Heat the olive oil in a saucepan. Add the turkey, chili powder, salt, pepper, and cumin and sauté and saute for 7 to 8 minutes, chopping often with the spatula, until the turkey is cooked through.

2. Add the onion and sauté for 1 minute more before adding the cilantro, beans with liquid, and chicken stock. Bring to a boil, and minimize the heat to low, cover, and let simmer for 15 minutes. Divide between 4 soup bowls and serve hot.

EGGPLANT, HUMMUS, AND GOAT CHEESE SANDWICHES

Grilled slices of eggplant replace deli meats, and hummus adds protein and fiber while taking the place of mayonnaise. Try this classic Greek recipe and bring a Mediterranean flair to your lunch table.

Ingredients

- 1 medium eggplant, sliced ½ inch thick
- Sea salt
- 2 tablespoons olive oil
- Freshly ground black pepper
- 5 to 6 tablespoons hummus
- 4 slices whole wheat bread, toasted
- 1 cup baby spinach leaves
- 2 ounces goat cheese or feta cheese, softened

Preparations

1. Preheat a gas or charcoal grill to medium-high heat.
2. Add salt to each sides of the eggplant that has been sliced, and let it sit for few minutes to drain out the bitter juices. Rinse the eggplant and dry with a paper towel.
3. Brush the eggplant with the olive oil then season to taste with salt and pepper.
4. Grill the eggplant until lightly charred on both sides but still slightly firm in the middle, 3 to 4 minutes per side.
5. Spread the hummus on 2 Slices of the bread and top with the spinach leaves, goat cheese, and eggplant. Top with the rest of the slices of bread and serve warm.

VEGETABLE MARKET SCRAMBLE

There's nothing wrong with breakfast for lunch. This dish cooks up in just a few Minutes and will keep you going all day long.

Ingredients

- 1 teaspoon olive oil
- ½ red bell pepper, diced
- ½ cup diced white onion
- 1 cup sliced fresh mushrooms
- ½ teaspoon salt
- ¼ teaspoon freshly ground black pepper
- 8 large eggs, beaten

Preparations

1. Heat the olive oil in a skillet. Add the bell pepper, onion, mushrooms, salt, and pepper and sauté for 5 minutes, stirring frequently.
2. Pour the eggs over all and scramble, stirring constantly, for about 3 minutes, or until the eggs are set. Divide between 4 plates and serve hot.

DINNER

The recipes for non-fasting days are low in calories but suitable for guests or the entire family, so we've created most of them to make four servings. If you like, you can either halve the ingredients or freeze extra servings for easy reheating on another day.

TANGY ORANGE CHICKEN BREAST

This recipe delivers on both speed and flavor. It's a terrific dish to whip up on busy nights. Served with a green salad and some quinoa or brown rice, it's a light but satisfying Meal.

Ingredients

- 1 teaspoon olive oil
- 4 (4-to 5-ounce) skinless chicken breasts
- 1 teaspoon paprika
- ½ teaspoon salt
- ¼ teaspoon freshly ground black pepper
- 1 teaspoon chopped fresh thyme
- 1 teaspoon chopped fresh rosemary
- 1 tablespoon unsweetened orange juice concentrate
- 2 tablespoons chopped fresh parsley

Preparations

1. Preheat the oven to 400° F and line a baking dish with aluminum foil. Spread the olive oil all over the bottom of the dish.
2. Place the chicken breasts in the dish, flip over to coat with oil, and season with the paprika, salt, pepper, thyme, and rosemary.
3. Bake for 20 minutes, and flip the chicken and brush with the orange juice concentrate. Bake for 15 to 20 minutes more, or until the chicken juices run clear.
4. Garnish with the parsley before serving.

GRILLED SHRIMP AND BLACK BEAN SALAD

This recipe is the best one to use when you have company for dinner. No one will think it's low-calorie!

Ingredients

- 1 teaspoon lime zest (about ½ lime)
- ¼ cup freshly squeezed lime juice
- 3 tablespoons olive oil
- 2 tablespoons chopped fresh basil
- 2 tablespoons chopped fresh oregano
- 1 teaspoon freshly ground black pepper
- ½ teaspoon salt
- 2 cans black beans, washed and drained
- 1 cup diced tomatoes
- 1 cup diced green bell pepper
- ½ cup chopped green onions
- 24 large (21–25 Count) raw shrimp, peeled and deveined

Preparation

1. In a medium bowl, combine the juice and lime zest, olive oil, basil, oregano, and pepper and mix well. Measure 2 tablespoons out into a small bowl and set aside.
2. Add the salt, black beans, tomatoes, bell pepper, and onions to the medium bowl and toss well. Place in the refrigerator until serving.

3. Preheat a flat grill over medium-high heat. Once hot, place the shrimp on the grill and baste with the reserved lime juice mixture. Cook for about five mins on one side and then turn, baste again, and cook for 3 minutes more.
4. To serve, place one-quarter of the bean salad onto each plate and top with 6 hot shrimp.

MUSTARD-MAPLE-GLAZED SALMON

This is an incredibly delicious recipe for salmon, especially given how quick and simple it is to prepare. Add some brown rice or a baked sweet potato and you have a flavorful, rich Meal.

Ingredients

- 4 (6-ounce) skin-on salmon fillets, ¾ inch thick
- 1 teaspoon olive oil
- ½ teaspoon salt
- ½ teaspoon freshly ground black pepper
- 2 tablespoons pure maple syrup
- ½ teaspoon dry mustard
- 8 sprigs fresh thyme

Preparation

1. Preheat a flat grill over medium-high heat.

2. Brush the salmon fillets on each sides with the olive oil, season with pepper and salt, and put them all skin side down on the grill. Cook for 7 minutes.
3. Meanwhile, combine the maple syrup and dry mustard with a fork.
4. Flip the salmon fillets, brush with the maple-mustard glaze, and top each one with 2 Sprigs of the thyme. Grill for 5 to 10 minutes more, or until the fish flakes easily.
5. To serve, make use of a spatula to transfer the fillets to 4 plates, leaving the thyme intact.

TUSCAN-STYLE BAKED SEA BASS

Sea bass is a tasty fish—fine and flaky. This Tuscan-inspired recipe complements this Mild fish with the flavors of fresh tomatoes, walnuts, basil, and garlic.

Ingredients

- 4 (6-ounce) skin-on sea bass fillets
- 1 teaspoon olive oil
- 1 cup very finely chopped walnuts (use processor or blender)
- 2 teaspoons minced garlic
- 8 slices yellow or orange tomatoes, ¼ inch thick
- 8 slices red onion, ¼ inch thick
- ½ cup chopped fresh basil
- ½ teaspoon salt
- ¼ teaspoon freshly ground black pepper

Preparation

1. Preheat the oven to $400°F$ and line a baking sheet with aluminum foil.
2. Brush both sides of the bass fillets with the olive oil and then dip in the chopped walnuts, covering the fillets fully. Put the fillets skin all side down on the baking sheet. Spread the garlic over the fillets, then cover the fish with alternating tomato and onion slices. Spray the basil on top and season with pepper and salt.
3. Bake for 12 to 14 minutes, or until the fish flakes easily. To serve, make use of a spatula to transfer the fillets to 4 plates.

PORTOBELLO CHEESEBURGERS

It's not necessary you are a vegetarian to love these burgers, Made with succulent portobello mushrooms. They're deliciously different but every bit as satisfying as a traditional burger, without all the fat and calories. Cannellini beans tucked under the caps make them filling enough for even the hungriest eater.

Ingredients

- 4 large (4 inches wide) portobello mushroom caps
- 1½ teaspoons olive oil, divided
- ½ teaspoon salt
- ¼ teaspoon freshly ground black pepper
- ½ teaspoon minced garlic
- ½ teaspoon paprika
- 1 cup canned cannellini beans
- 4 (1-ounce) slices reduced-fat mozzarella cheese
- 4 whole wheat hamburger buns
- 4 large leaves romaine lettuce
- 4 slices fresh tomato
- 8 slices red onion

Preparation

1. Preheat the oven to 325 degrees F.
2. Rub the cap sides of the mushrooms with ½ teaspoon of the olive oil and season with salt and pepper.
3. In a skillet, heat the remaining 1 teaspoon olive oil over medium-high heat. Add the mushrooms, cap side down, and sauté for 4 minutes.
4. Meanwhile, mix together the garlic, paprika, and beans and heat in the microwave for 1 minute, or just until warm. Set aside.
5. Flip the mushrooms and place 1 slice of mozzarella onto each one. Reduce the heat to low.
6. Toast the hamburger buns in the oven for 5 minutes, or just until crisp. Transfer to 4 plates. Top the bottom buns with the tomato, lettuce, and onion.

7. Spoon one-quarter of the bean mixture into a mound in the center of each bun and top with a mushroom, cap side up. Add the top buns and serve.

FLANK STEAK SPINACH SALAD

Flank steak is a flavorful and lean cut of Meat that is ideal for a low-calorie diet. This recipe calls for the steak to be cooked medium rare. The Meat tends to get quite tough if cooked much more than that.

Ingredients

- 1 pound flank steak, visible fat and sinew removed
- ¼ cup Balsamic Vinaigrette, divided
- ½ teaspoon salt
- ½ teaspoon freshly ground black pepper
- 3 Cups chopped romaine lettuce
- 1 cup baby spinach leaves
- 1 pint cherry tomatoes, halved
- ½ cup thinly sliced sweet yellow onion

Preparation

1. Preheat a flat grill over high heat until it is very hot.

2. Brush the flank steak with 2 tablespoons of the Balsamic Vinaigrette, season with the salt and pepper, and place on the grill. Cook for few minutes, flip and cook for 10 minutes more, or until the steak is medium rare.
3. Meanwhile, combine the lettuce, spinach, tomatoes, and onion until well mixed. Then add the remaining 2 tablespoons vinaigrette dressing. Toss well to coat and divide the salad between 4 plates.
4. Transfer the flank steak to a plate and allow it to rest for 10 minutes before slicing thinly on the diagonal.
5. Place one-quarter of the sliced steak on top of each salad and serve.

CHICKEN PICADILLO

This variation on a traditional Latin dish uses leaner chicken in place of beef. It takes nothing away from the zesty flavor, but it does reduce the fat and calories usually present in the traditional version. Make an extra ration to freeze for later.

Ingredients

- 2 teaspoons olive oil
- ½ cup chopped yellow onion
- 2 Cloves garlic, chopped
- ½ pound ground chicken
- ½ teaspoon ground cumin
- ½ teaspoon salt
- ¼ teaspoon freshly ground black pepper

- 2 tablespoons red wine
- 1 cup chopped tomato
- 1 fresh jalapeño pepper, seeded and diced
- ¼ cup green olives with pimientos, chopped
- 1 teaspoon Worcestershire sauce
- ¼ cup chopped fresh cilantro
- 1 teaspoon fresh lime juice (about ½ lime)

Preparation

1. Heat the olive oil in a skillet. Add the garlic and onion then sauté for 2 minutes, stirring often.
2. Add the chicken, cumin, salt, and pepper and cook for 5 to 6 minutes, stirring frequently to crumble the chicken.
3. Add the wine into the pan to deglaze it, scraping any browned bits from the bottom. Add the tomato, jalapeño, olives, and Worcestershire sauce; reduce the heat to medium and let simmer for 8 minutes, or until the mixture has thickened.
4. To serve, ladle into 4 bowls and finish with a squeeze of lime and a sprinkling of cilantro.

CHICKEN FLORENTINE-STYLE

In this riff on true Florentine dishes, chicken breasts are treated with a delicious creamy sauce studded with fresh spinach. Serve this one to your guests—they'll have no idea you're on a diet.

Ingredients

- 1 teaspoon olive oil
- 4 (6-ounce) boneless skinless chicken breasts
- ½ teaspoon salt
- ¼ teaspoon freshly ground black pepper
- ¼ cup dry white wine
- ¼ cup chopped yellow onion
- 1 cup sliced fresh mushrooms
- 1 cup ice-covered chopped spinach, defrosted and drained
- ½ cup chicken stock
- ¼ cup low-fat milk
- ¼ cup shredded Parmesan cheese

Preparation

1. Heat the olive oil in a skillet.
2. Season the chicken breasts on each sides with the salt and pepper and sauté for 5 minutes. Flip the chicken and cook for 5 to 7 minutes more, or until the juices run clear. Transfer to a plate then cover it to keep warm.
3. Add the wine to the pan to deglaze it, and scrape up any browned bits from the bottom.
4. Add the onion, mushrooms, spinach, and chicken stock, and simmer for 10 to 15 minutes, or until the sauce is reduced by half.
5. Decrease the heat, stir in the milk, and heat just until warmed though, about 1 minute.

6. To serve, put one chicken breast on each plate, top with one-quarter of the sauce, and sprinkle with the Parmesan cheese.

EASY BLACK BEAN SOUP

When served with a fresh salad and a crusty roll, this dish is a comforting and filling Meal. You'll get all the flavors of traditional black bean soup but in far less time.

Ingredients

- 2 (15-ounce) cans black beans
- ½ teaspoon chili powder
- 2 Cups chicken stock
- 1 cup thinly sliced carrots
- ½ cup chopped yellow onion
- ½ teaspoon garlic powder
- ½ teaspoon ground cumin
- ½ teaspoon salt
- ¼ teaspoon freshly ground black pepper
- 1 cup plain yogurt
- ¼ cup sliced green onions

Preparation

1. Over medium heat, mix the black beans, chicken stock, carrots, onion, garlic powder, cumin, chili powder, and salt in a saucepan. Stir well.
2. Boil the soup, reduce the heat to medium, cover, and simmer for 20 minutes, stirring occasionally.
3. To serve, ladle into 4 bowls, top with a large dollop of yogurt, and garnish with green onions.

HEARTY VEGETABLE SOUP

The vegetable soup is very easy to make and is just packed with a wide variety of vegetables. It's a great soup to serve alongside a salad or sandwich on those nights when you don't feel like cooking, so double up and freeze the extra.

Ingredients

- 1 teaspoon olive oil
- 1 cup diced Yukon Gold potatoes
- ½ cup thinly sliced carrots
- ½ cup fresh green beans, slice into 1-inch pieces
- ½ cup chopped yellow onion
- 1 cup fresh spinach leaves
- 3 Cups chicken stock
- ¼ cup chopped fresh parsley
- 1 tablespoon chopped fresh rosemary
- ½ teaspoon salt
- ¼ teaspoon freshly ground black pepper

Preparation

1. Heat the olive oil in a skillet. Add the potatoes, carrots, green beans, and onion and sauté for 5 minutes, stirring frequently. Remove from the heat.
2. Transfer the vegetables to a large saucepan over medium-high heat. Add the spinach, chicken stock, parsley, rosemary, salt, and pepper and bring the soup to a boil. Reduce the heat, cover it, then simmer for 30 minutes.
3. To serve, ladle into 4 bowls.

MUSHROOM-STUFFED ZUCCHINI

Fresh zucchini and mushrooms Seasoned with garlic, olive oil, parsley, and Italian herbs and spices hardly seems like diet food. These mushroom-stuffed zucchini boats Make an easy and impressive dish that is low in calories but still plenty filling. Serve with a piece of fish for dinner, or serve alone for lunch.

Ingredients

- 2 tablespoons olive oil
- 2 Cups finely chopped button mushrooms
- 2 Cloves garlic, finely chopped
- 2 tablespoons chicken stock
- 1 tablespoon finely chopped flat-leaf parsley
- 1 tablespoon Italian seasoning

- Sea salt
- Freshly ground black pepper
- 2 medium zucchini, cut in half lengthwise
- 1 tablespoon water

Preparation

1. Preheat the oven to 350 degrees F.
2. Heat a skillet, then add put in olive oil. Add the mushrooms, allow it to cook until tender, about 4 minutes. Add the garlic and cook for 2 minutes more. Add the chicken then cook for four minutes more.
3. Add the parsley and Italian seasoning, then season with salt and pepper to taste. Stir well and remove from the heat.
4. Scoop out some of the flesh and the seeds of the halved zucchini and stuff the halves with the mushroom mixture.
5. Put the zucchini inside a casserole dish, and drizzle 1 tablespoon water in the bottom.
6. Cover with aluminum foil and bake for 30 to 40 minutes, or until the zucchini boats are tender. Transfer to 2 plates and serve immediately.

ZESTY BEEF KABOBS

Tender, juicy, and zesty, these kabobs are going to Make you glad you're eating healthy. Yet more proof that eating lean doesn't have to taste unappetizing!

Ingredients

- ½ cup lime juice
- 1 teaspoon salt
- 1 teaspoon black pepper
- 1 clove garlic, minced
- ¼ teaspoon red pepper flakes
- ¼ teaspoon rosemary, chopped
- ¼ teaspoon basil, chopped
- 1 pound lean red meat, such as beef, venison, or bison, chunked into bitesized cubes
- 1 red onion, peeled, cut in half horizontally, and quartered vertically
- 1 pack cherry tomatoes
- 2 green peppers, cut similarly to the onion

Preparation

1. Mix together the first seven ingredients.
2. Add meat to a large plastic zip bag, and pour the lime and spice mixture over it. Marinate for at least 20 minutes—the longer the better.
3. Preheat grill to medium/high when you're ready to make the kabobs. Thread the meat, onions, tomatoes, and peppers onto your skewers.
4. Grill 1–3 minutes on each of the four sides, or until your steak reaches desired temp.

CONCLUSION

To change a healthy lifestyle, it takes determination and commitment. Adjusting to a healthy diet with whole foods can be overwhelming, especially if you are following a typical Western diet full of ready-made meals, fast food, and high-sugar treats.

However, the change in your body, your energy levels, and the way you feel after a few weeks of the Fast 5: 2 diet will make all of your hard work worth it. Many individuals report that they feel much more energetic and focused after just a week or two. If you aim to lose weight and excess body fat, you will likely see results within the first week.

More importantly, the changes you make to your diet, along with regular physical activity, will more than make you feel better and look slimmer. They will contribute to your overall health and can help prevent many of the diet-related illnesses and conditions we see today.

While your good looks are your reward, the importance of positively impacting the length and quality of your life cannot be overstated.

So when you're tempted by old eating habits or the occasional craving, grab a healthy snack and re-read the motivational tips we offer, take a long walk, or invite a friend to join you for one of your scheduled treats.

Remembering the reasons you do what you do and celebrating how you look and feel can provide you with the energy required to overcome the obstacles on your way to better health.

Manufactured by Amazon.ca
Acheson, AB